Preventing Suicide in Patients with Mental Disorders

Preventing Suicide in Patients with Mental Disorders

Editors

**Maurizio Pompili
Andrea Fiorillo**

MDPI • Basel • Beijing • Wuhan • Barcelona • Belgrade • Manchester • Tokyo • Cluj • Tianjin

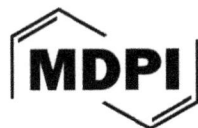

Editors
Maurizio Pompili
Sapienza University of Rome
Italy

Andrea Fiorillo
University of Campania "L. Vanvitelli"
Italy

Editorial Office
MDPI
St. Alban-Anlage 66
4052 Basel, Switzerland

This is a reprint of articles from the Special Issue published online in the open access journal *Medicina* (ISSN 1010-660X) (available at: https://www.mdpi.com/journal/medicina/special_issues/Preventing_Suicide_Patients_Mental_Disorders).

For citation purposes, cite each article independently as indicated on the article page online and as indicated below:

LastName, A.A.; LastName, B.B.; LastName, C.C. Article Title. *Journal Name* **Year**, *Article Number*, Page Range.

ISBN 978-3-03943-677-4 (Hbk)
ISBN 978-3-03943-678-1 (PDF)

© 2020 by the authors. Articles in this book are Open Access and distributed under the Creative Commons Attribution (CC BY) license, which allows users to download, copy and build upon published articles, as long as the author and publisher are properly credited, which ensures maximum dissemination and a wider impact of our publications.

The book as a whole is distributed by MDPI under the terms and conditions of the Creative Commons license CC BY-NC-ND.

Contents

About the Editors vii

Preface to "Preventing Suicide in Patients with Mental Disorders" ix

Giovanna Fico, Vito Caivano, Francesca Zinno, Marco Carfagno, Luca Steardo Jr., Gaia Sampogna, Mario Luciano and Andrea Fiorillo
Affective Temperaments and Clinical Course of Bipolar Disorder: An Exploratory Study of Differences among Patients with and without a History of Violent Suicide Attempts
Reprinted from: *Medicina* **2019**, *55*, 390, doi:10.3390/medicina55070390 1

Marco Paolini, David Lester, Michael Hawkins, Ameth Hawkins-Villarreal, Denise Erbuto, Andrea Fiorillo and Maurizio Pompili
Cytomegalovirus Seropositivity and Suicidal Behavior: A Mini-Review
Reprinted from: *Medicina* **2019**, *55*, 782, doi:10.3390/medicina55120782 13

Carla Gramaglia, Raffaella Calati and Patrizia Zeppegno
Rational Suicide in Late Life: A Systematic Review of the Literature
Reprinted from: *Medicina* **2019**, *55*, 656, doi:10.3390/medicina55100656 23

Alessandra Costanza, Massimo Prelati and Maurizio Pompili
The Meaning in Life in Suicidal Patients: The Presence and the Search for Constructs. A Systematic Review
Reprinted from: *Medicina* **2019**, *55*, 465, doi:10.3390/medicina55080465 47

Luca Bonanni, Flavia Gualtieri, David Lester, Giulia Falcone, Adele Nardella, Andrea Fiorillo and Maurizio Pompili
Can Anhedonia Be Considered a Suicide Risk Factor? A Review of the Literature
Reprinted from: *Medicina* **2019**, *55*, 458, doi:10.3390/medicina55080458 65

Peter Dome, Zoltan Rihmer and Xenia Gonda
Suicide Risk in Bipolar Disorder: A Brief Review
Reprinted from: *Medicina* **2019**, *55*, 403, doi:10.3390/medicina55080403 79

Leo Sher and René S. Kahn
Suicide in Schizophrenia: An Educational Overview
Reprinted from: *Medicina* **2019**, *55*, 361, doi:10.3390/medicina55070361 87

Joel Paris
Suicidality in Borderline Personality Disorder
Reprinted from: *Medicina* **2019**, *55*, 223, doi:10.3390/medicina55060223 99

Isabella Berardelli, Salvatore Sarubbi, Elena Rogante, Michael Hawkins, Gabriele Cocco, Denise Erbuto, David Lester and Maurizio Pompili
The Role of Demoralization and Hopelessness in Suicide Risk in Schizophrenia: A Review of the Literature
Reprinted from: *Medicina* **2019**, *55*, 200, doi:10.3390/medicina55050200 105

Mark Schechter, Elsa Ronningstam, Benjamin Herbstman and Mark J. Goldblatt
Psychotherapy with Suicidal Patients: The Integrative Psychodynamic Approach of the Boston Suicide Study Group
Reprinted from: *Medicina* **2019**, *55*, 303, doi:10.3390/medicina55060303 123

About the Editors

Maurizio Pompili (M.D., Ph.D.) is a Full Professor and Chair of Psychiatry as part of the Faculty of Medicine and Psychology at Sapienza University of Rome, Italy, where he received his M.D. degree, where he trained in Psychiatry (both summa cum laude). He is the Director of the Residency Training Program in Psychiatry of his faculty. He is the Director of the University Psychiatric Clinic and the Director of the Suicide Prevention Center at Sant'Andrea Hospital in Rome.

He is the President of the Psychiatric Rehabilitation Technique degree program at the Sapienza University of Rome.

He has a doctoral degree in Experimental and Clinical Neurosciences. He was also part of the Community at McLean Hospital—Harvard Medical School, the USA, where he received a psychiatry fellowship.

He is the recipient of the American Association of Suicidology's 2008 Shneidman Award for "Outstanding contributions in research in suicidology."

Apart from being the Italian Representative of the International Association for Suicide Prevention (IASP) for eight years, he has was also one of the Vice-Presidents of this association. He is now a Co-Chair of the IASP Special Interest Group in Risk Resilience and Reasons for Living. He is also a member of the International Academy for Suicide Research and the American Association of Suicidology. He is also President of the Suicidology Section of the Italian Psychiatric Society.

He has published more than 400 papers on suicide, bipolar disorders, and other psychiatric perspectives, including original research articles, book chapters, and editorials. He co-edited ten international books on suicide.

He ranks in the top 10 suicide authors of 500 world suicide authors listed in the ISI Web of Science (this is in terms of the number of focused works on the topic of suicide that are indexed in the ISI Web of Science).

He has been recognized by Expertscape as an expert in suicide, ranking 1st worldwide. H-index: 54 (October 2020).

Andrea Fiorillo (M.D., Ph.D.) is a Full Professor of Psychiatry in Naples (Italy) at the University of Campania "L. Vanvitelli".

He is currently a Board member of the European Psychiatric Association (EPA) and Secretary for Scientific Sections. He is the Chair of the Section on Education in Psychiatry of the World Psychiatric Association (WPA), a member of the WPA Operational Committee on Education, Honorary Member of the WPA, and President of the Italian Society for Social Psychiatry.

He is the Editor-in-Chief of *European Psychiatry*. He has authored about 250 scientific papers in international peer-reviewed journals. He has edited more than 10 books and several chapters in the field of mental health. He has extensively lectured abroad. His main research interests include clinical and social psychiatry, academic psychiatry, psychiatric epidemiology, prevention of mental disorders, and promotion of physical and mental health in people with severe mental illnesses.

Preface to "Preventing Suicide in Patients with Mental Disorders"

Suicide is a multi-factorial, highly prevalent clinical condition; it is estimated that every 30 seconds a person worldwide commits suicide. Moreover, it represents the second most common cause of death in adolescents, and it is a major health problem, which requires the development and adoption of appropriate preventive strategies.

Suicide is a complex phenomenon that is now considered understood as a neurodevelopmental condition encompassing childhood experiences and proximal conditions, such as mental disorders and adverse life events. Individuals in crisis may face overwhelming psychological pain, which in some cases may overcome the threshold of each unique individual for whom suicide is considered the best option to deal with such pain. However, many socio-demographic, personal, or temperamental variables have been investigated for their causal association with suicide risk, but, to date, no single factor has clearly demonstrated an association with suicide. The mental disorders most frequently associated with suicide risk include bipolar disorders and major unipolar depression, substance use disorders, and schizophrenia. However, anxiety, personality, eating, and trauma-related disorders, as well as organic mental disorders, also contribute to suicidal risk. Moreover, in modern society, the presence of social uncertainty, changes in family models, development of social media, and loss of face-to-face interaction can have an impact on suicide risk, particularly in the younger generation.

We are pleased to invite you and your co-workers to contribute to this Special Issue with original research reports, reviews, or meta-analyses on the topics of suicide and mental disorders, the social and personal burden of suicide, and the possible preventive strategies to be implemented for reducing suicidal risk for each mental disorder considered. All mental disorders as well as mental health problems associated with an increased risk of suicide can be considered for publication in this Special Issue.

Maurizio Pompili, Andrea Fiorillo
Editors

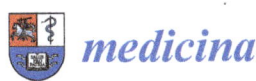

Article

Affective Temperaments and Clinical Course of Bipolar Disorder: An Exploratory Study of Differences among Patients with and without a History of Violent Suicide Attempts

Giovanna Fico [1,*], Vito Caivano [1], Francesca Zinno [1], Marco Carfagno [1], Luca Steardo Jr. [2], Gaia Sampogna [1], Mario Luciano [1] and Andrea Fiorillo [1]

1 Department of Psychiatry, University of Campania "L. Vanvitelli", Largo Madonna Delle Grazie, 80139 Naples, Italy
2 Department of Health Sciences, Psychiatric Unit, University Magna Graecia of Catanzaro, Viale Europa, 88100 Catanzaro CZ, Italy
* Correspondence: giov.fico@gmail.com; Tel.: +39-081-5666531; Fax: +39-081-5666523

Received: 11 June 2017; Accepted: 15 July 2019; Published: 19 July 2019

Abstract: *Background and Objectives:* Suicide is the leading cause of death in patients with Bipolar Disorder (BD). In particular, the high mortality rate is due to violent suicide attempts. Several risk factors associated with suicide attempts in patients with BD have been identified. Affective temperaments are associated with suicidal risk, but their predictive role is still understudied. The aim of this study is to assess the relationship between affective temperaments and personal history of violent suicide attempts. *Materials and Methods:* 74 patients with Bipolar Disorder type I (BD-I) or II (BD-II) were included. All patients filled in the short version of Munster Temperament Evaluation of the Memphis, Pisa, Paris and San Diego (short TEMPS-M) and the Temperament and Character Inventory, revised version (TCI-R). The sample was divided into two groups on the basis of a positive history for suicidal attempts and the suicidal group was further divided into two subgroups according to violent suicide attempts. *Results:* Violent suicide attempts were positively associated with the cyclothymic temperament and inversely to the hyperthymic one. BD-I patients and patients with a clinical history of rapid cycling were significantly more represented in the group of patients with a history of violent suicide attempts. *Conclusions:* Our study highlights that several clinical and temperamental characteristics are associated with violent suicide attempts, suggesting the importance of affective temperaments in the clinical management of patients with BPI.

Keywords: bipolar; suicide; affective temperament; violent suicide; aggressive behaviors

1. Introduction

According to the World Health Organization (WHO), suicide is one of the leading causes of death worldwide accounting for nearly 800,000 deaths every year [1]. Psychiatric disorders are an important contributing factor to suicide attempts [2] and bipolar disorders (BDs) are associated with the highest suicide risk [3], which is 15–30 times higher than the general population. Up to one-half of patients with BDs attempt suicide in their lifetime [4].

Suicide is a complex and multivariate phenomenon, defined as "death caused by self-directed injurious behavior with intent to die" [5] which can be performed by several means, including violent and non-violent methods. Suicide methods are noteworthy to be characterized, since they can contribute defining a suicidal subpopulation more vulnerable to suicide completion. In fact, violent suicide attempters have been proved to have an elevated risk of future suicide attempts [6], as well as a higher immediate lethality of an attempt [7] with a fatality rate over 70% [8]. Although a violent suicide attempt is usually defined by the method, there is no clear consensus about its definition. Asberg [9] identifies a few violent attempts (i.e., hanging, gas poisoning and drowning), whereas drug overdoses are considered to be non-violent suicide attempts. Subsequently, Giner (2014) [10] and Penas-Lledo (2015) [11] adopted and extended Asberg's criteria by including in the definition of "violent attempts" the use of firearms, jumping from heights, several deep cuts, car crash, burning, electrocution, and jumping under a train. Likewise, Dumais (2005) [12] enlarges the list of non-violent suicide attempts by adding drowning and gas poisoning. The identification of a subpopulation, such as the violent suicide attempters, of patients with mental disorders at higher risk to commit suicide and the identification of the risk factors of suicide attempts is a stepping stone in the development of a better suicide prevention strategy.

Several risk factors linked to suicide attempts in patients with BD have been identified in previous studies, including a long duration of illness, untreated BD, female sex, positive history for suicide attempts, comorbidity with substance abuse or personality disorders, anxiety, depressive polarity [13], recent affective episodes, and recent psychiatric inpatient care [14]. Personality and temperamental traits have also been considered, and anger, impulsivity, aggression, anxiety and two factors (i.e., "harm avoidance" and "novelty seeking") of the Temperament and Character Inventory (TCI) have been identified to be associated with suicide attempts [15]. Only recently temperament and, in particular, affective temperaments have been considered as possible factors linked to suicide attempts [16]. Temperament represents the "temporally stable biological core of personality" affecting several aspects of an individual's life (activity level, rhythms, moods and related cognitions) while personality, a broader phenotype, also refers to "acquired characterological determinants and interpersonal operations" [16]. Akiskal et al. conceptualized a *spectrum* of *affective* conditions ranging from *temperament* to clinical episodes [17] and proposed criteria defining five temperaments: (1) Cyclothymic temperament, characterized by chronic cycling between mood polarities and unstable self-esteem and energy; (2) hyperthymic temperament, characterized by increased energy and optimism [17]; (3) irritable temperament, characterized by irritable and angry behavior; (4) anxious temperament, characterized by a tendency to worry; (5) depressive temperament, characterized by low levels of energy, introversion and worrying [18]. Affective temperaments, conceptualized as stable, subclinical forms of the manic-depressive illness by Akiskal (1983), have a role in the clinical evolution of the mood disorders and the outcome, including the risk of suicide attempts [19]. In particular, hyperthymic temperament has been shown to be associated with a reduced risk of suicide attempts [20,21], whereas cyclothymic, irritable, depressive and anxious temperaments are more present in patients with a positive history of suicide attempts [22,23]. Besides, cyclothymic and irritable temperaments are highly connected with both aggression [24] and impulsivity [25], which play a role in suicidal behavior. A widely used questionnaire to evaluate affective temperaments is the Temperament Evaluation of Memphis, Pisa, Paris and San Diego (TEMPS) [18,26] which has been developed in different formats and used in clinical and research settings [27]. It has been documented that affective temperaments individually considered, have reduced predictive power if used to anticipate suicidal risk [28], while composite TEMPS-A score yields stronger associations with suicidal risk and better identify subjects at risk for suicide attempts [20]. A few data on the clinical characteristics of violent attempters with BDs are available. Existing data suggest that violent attempters are more likely to be men [29], have the first episode of manic/hypomanic type [30] and carry the serotonin transporter gene S allele [31].

To our knowledge, there are no previous studies that specifically addressed the issue of the association between affective temperament subtypes and a history of violent suicide attempts in BDs. Thus, the aim of our study is to investigate the relationship between affective temperaments and personal history of violent suicide attempts, defined according to Asberg's criteria, in a clinical sample of bipolar patients.

2. Materials and Methods

The exploratory study was carried out in the bipolar outpatient unit of the Department of Psychiatry of the University of Campania "Luigi Vanvitelli", in Naples between January and June 2018. The only inclusion criterion was a diagnosis of bipolar disorder type I or II according to the DSM 5 criteria. Patients were excluded if they have presented affective illness as a consequence of alcohol/substance abuse or dependence, medical illness, an organic brain disorder or medication, and if not able to provide written informed consent (i.e., dementia, cognitive impairment or delirium). The study was approved by the local ethical review board (N001567/28.01.2018).

All patients filled in the short version of the Munster Temperament Evaluation of the Memphis, Pisa, Paris and San Diego (short TEMPS-M) [32,33], a 35 items questionnaire used to assess affective temperaments described by Akiskal (depressive, anxious, hyperthymic, cyclothymic and irritable) using a dimensional approach with a five-point Likert type scale ranging from 1 to 5 (1 = "not at all"; 2 = "a little"; 3 = "moderately"; 4 = "much"; 5 "very much") [34] and the Temperament and Character Inventory, revised version (TCI-R) [35]. The TCI was developed by Cloninger, with the goal of assessing factors underlying the psychobiological aspect of personality. The revised version (TCI-R) is a questionnaire consisting of 240 items, with a 5-point Likert-type scale, grouped into four temperament dimensions, novelty seeking (NS), harm avoidance (HA), reward dependence (RD) and persistence (PS), and three character dimensions, self-directiveness (SD), cooperativeness (CO) and self-transcendence (ST) samples [36].

Patients' and clinicians' socio-demographic and clinical characteristics were analyzed using descriptive and frequency counts, as appropriate. The sample was divided into two groups on the basis of a positive history for a suicidal attempt. Differences among groups were evaluated using χ^2 or Bonferroni-adjusted T-test, as appropriate. Suicidal patients were further divided into two subgroups according to the history of violent suicide attempts, in line with Asberg's criteria (1976). A logistic multivariable regression model was performed in order to identify factors associated with a positive history of suicidal behavior. All possible confounders were entered in the model. Statistical analyses were performed using SPSS version 18, the level of statistical significance was set at the level of $p < 0.05$.

3. Results

The sample consists of 74 patients. Patients' sociodemographic characteristics, as well as patients' clinical features, are reported in Table 1. The sample is composed by 36 men (48.7%) and 38 women (51.3%), with a mean age of 48.92 years (SD = 12.38), the most frequent diagnosis was bipolar II disorder (59.5%). The samples grouped according to a positive history of suicide attempts (Table 2). Forty patients have a positive history of suicide attempts (45.9%). Psychotic symptoms are more frequent in patients with a history of suicide attempts compared to patients without a history of suicide attempts ($p < 0.019$), and particularly during mixed episodes ($p < 0.008$). Furthermore, suicidal attempters show a higher rate of aggressive behaviors, but no differences were found between the two groups in terms of the clinical course of the disease, number of psychiatric admissions, number of affective episodes and seasonality. Depressive, anxious and cyclothymic temperaments are more represented in suicidal attempters, while hyperthymic in non-suicidal ones. Suicidal attempters have been further divided into two subgroups according to violent suicide attempts in line with Asberg's criteria (Table 3). Twenty-four patients report a history of violent suicide attempts, 54.2% being females and 45.8% males with a mean age of 49.46 (SD = 13.02); the most frequent diagnosis is BDI (75%); 41.7% of violent attempters and 45.83% of non-violent attempters were on lithium therapy. A clinical course of rapid cycling (4 or more affective episodes during a year) is significantly more represented in the group of patients with a history of violent suicide attempts. Furthermore, violent attempters show a higher rate of cyclothymic temperament and lower rates of hyperthymic temperament. At the multivariate logistic regression, we found that the hyperthymic temperament reduces the likelihood to have a positive history of suicidal attempts ($p < 0.01$) (Table 4).

Table 1. Socio-demographic and clinical characteristics of the sample (N = 74).

Gender, male (N; %)	(36; 48.6)
Diagnosis, Bipolar disorder type I (N; %)	(30; 40.5%)
Age (mean ± SD)	(48.92 ± 12.38)
Age at illness onset (mean ± SD)	(27.71 ± 9.8)
Duration of illness (mean ± SD)	(16.07 ± 9.46)
Number of depressive episodes (mean ± SD)	(7.1 ± 5.22)
Number of manic episodes (mean ± SD)	(3.79 ± 2.06)
Number of hypomanic episodes (mean ± SD)	(6.48 ± 4.5)
Number of mixed episodes (mean ± SD)	(2.53 ± 1.16)
Lifetime number of affective episodes (mean ± SD)	(14.17 ± 9.59)
Number of affective episodes during last year (mean ± SD)	(2.04 ± 2.28)
Lifetime number of psychiatric admissions (mean ± SD)	(0.493 ± 0.92)
Duration of psychiatric admissions (mean ± SD)	(0.7 ± 1.44)
Clinical Course (N; %)	
Mania–Depression–Interval (MDI)	(11; 14.9)
Depression–Mania–Interval (DMI)	(10; 13.5)
Mania–Interval–Depression (MID)	(8; 10.8)
Depression–Interval–Mania (DIM)	(3; 4.1)
Rapid cycling	(8; 10.8)
Irregular cycling	(25; 33.8)
History of suicide attempts (N; %)	(40; 54.1)
Presence of psychotic symptoms, yes (N; %)	(36; 49.3)
during depressive episodes	(13; 9.5)
during manic episodes	(7; 17.6)
during mixed episodes	(15; 20.3)
Aggressive behaviours (N; %)	(32; 43.2)
brief TEMPS-M subscores (mean ± SD)	
Depressive (dep)	(23.58 ± 5.93)
Cyclothymic (cyc)	(23.76 ± 7.1)
Irritable (irr)	(18.96 ± 7.59)
Anxious (anx)	(19.82 ± 6.3)
Hyperthymic (hyp)	(19.97 ± 6.3)

Table 2. Socio-demographic and clinical characteristics of the sample divided by history of suicide attempts.

Factors	Suicidal	Non-Suicidal
Cases (N; %)	40; 45.9%	34; 54.1%
Gender, male (N; %)	19; 47.5	17; 50
Diagnosis, Bipolar disorder type I, (N; %)	18; 45%	12; 30%
Age (mean ± SD)	49.53 ± 13.16	48.21 ± 11.56
Age at illness onset (mean ± SD)	26.76 ± 9.230	28.67 ± 10.45
Duration of illness (mean ± SD)	16.69 ± 8.92	15.34 ± 10.14
Number of depressive episodes (mean ± SD)	6.49 ± 3.55	7.82 ± 6.67
Number of manic episodes (mean ± SD)	3.93 ± 1.92	3.62 ± 2.24
Number of hypomanic episodes (mean ± SD)	5.61 ± 2.48	7.50 ± 5.96
Number of mixed episodes (mean ± SD)	2.55 ± 0.86	2.51 ± 1.45
Lifetime number of affective episodes (mean ± SD)	12.97 ± 5.92	15.59 ± 12.57
Number of affective episodes during last year (mean ± SD)	1.74 ± 0.68	2.39 ± 3.28
Lifetime number of psychiatric admissions (mean ± SD)	0.58 ± 1.07	0.38 ± 0.69
Duration of psychiatric admissions (mean ± SD)	0.800 ± 1.63	0.588 ± 1.2090

Table 2. Cont.

Factors	Suicidal	Non-Suicidal
Clinical Course (N; %)		
Mania–Depression–Interval (MDI)	6; 15	5; 14.7
Depression–Mania–Interval (DMI)	6; 15	4; 11.8
Mania–Interval–Depression (MID)	3; 7.5	5; 14.7
Depression–Interval–Mania (DIM)	2; 5	1; 2.9
Rapid cycling	2; 5	6; 17.6
Irregular cycling	12; 30	13; 38.2
Presence of psychotic symptoms, yes (N; %)	25; 62.5 *	11; 32.4
during depressive episodes	4; 10	3; 8.8
during manic episodes	8; 20	5; 14.7
during mixed episodes	13; 32.5 *	2; 5.9
Seasonality (N; %)	16; 40.0	15; 32.4
Aggressive behaviours (N; %)	21; 52.5 *	11; 32.3
brief TEMPS-M subscores (mean ± SD)		
Depressive (dep)	25 ± 5.54	21.91 ± 6.01
Cyclothymic (cyc)	25.7 ± 6.38	21.47 ± 7.3
Irritable (irr)	19.68 ± 7.86	18.12 ± 7.29
Anxious (anx)	21.33 ± 6.31	18.06 ± 5.9
Hyperthymic (hyp)	18.13 ± 6.38 *	22.15 ± 5.53
TCI-R subscores (mean ± SD)		
NS total score	107.04 ± 18.19	106.34 ± 17.20
HA total score	113.85 ± 23.03	107.44 ± 23.87
RD total score	99.61 ± 16.54	99.04 ± 16.54
PS total score	100.09 ± 26.47	109.6 ± 24.85
SD total score	115.4 ± 22.16	123.2 ± 21.72
C total score	122.8 ± 16.14	124.3 ± 20.93
ST total score	73.13 ± 17.75	71.27 ± 13.25

Abbreviations: novelty seeking (NS), harm avoidance (HA), reward dependence (RD) and persistence (PS), self-directiveness (SD), cooperativeness (CO) and self-transcendence (ST). * $p < 0.002$ (Bonferroni).

Table 3. Socio-demographic and clinical characteristics of patients with a history of violent suicide attempts (N = 24).

Gender, male (N; %)	11; 45.8
Diagnosis, Bipolar disorder type I, (N; %)	18; 75%
Age (mean ± SD)	49.46 ± 13.02
Age at illness onset (mean ± SD)	27. 09 ± 8.73
Duration of illness (mean ± SD)	15.94 ± 10.42
Number of depressive episodes (mean ± SD)	7.57 ± 5.89
Number of manic episodes (mean ± SD)	3.76 ± 1.94
Number of hypomanic episodes (mean ± SD)	7.01 ± 5.20
Number of mixed episodes (mean ± SD)	2.52 ± 1.19
Lifetime number of affective episodes (mean ± SD)	14.88 ± 11.01
Number of affective episodes during last year (mean ± SD)	2.23 ± 11.01
Lifetime number of psychiatric admissions (mean ± SD)	0.380 ± 0 .69
Duration of psychiatric admissions (mean ± SD)	0.56 ± 1.12
Clinical Course (N; %)	
Mania–Depression–Interval (MDI)	4; 16.7
Depression–Mania–Interval (DMI)	5; 20.8
Mania–Interval–Depression (MID)	3; 12.5
Depression–Interval–Mania (DIM)	1; 4.2
Rapid cycling	8; 33.3 *
Irregular cycling	7; 29.2

Table 3. Cont.

Presence of psychotic symptoms, yes (N; %)	13; 54.2
during depressive episodes	3; 12.5
during manic episodes	6; 25
during mixed episodes	4; 16.7
Aggressive behaviours (N; %)	17; 70.8
Lithium Therapy (N; %)	10; 41.7%
brief TEMPS-M subscores	
Depressive (dep)	24.04 ± 6.29
Cyclothymic (cyc)	27.6 ± 5.39 *
Irritable (irr)	18.58 ± 7.64
Anxious (anx)	20.54 ± 5.71
Hyperthymic (hyp)	17.25 ± 5.60 *
TCI-R subscores (mean ± SD)	
NS total score	103.91 ± 18.59
HA total score	112.70 ± 26
RD total score	99.31 ± 13.9
PS total score	101.6 ± 27.45
SD total score	119.25 ± 21.79
C total score	124.02 ± 16.06
ST total score	71.3 ± 18.75

Abbreviations: novelty seeking (NS), harm avoidance (HA), reward dependence (RD) and persistence (PS), self-directiveness (SD), cooperativeness (CO) and self-transcendence (ST). * $p < 0.002$ (Bonferroni).

Table 4. Multivariate logistic regression, dependent variable: suicidal behavior vs. non-suicidal behavior.

Number of subjects included on the analysis	46		
F (df)	4.816 (1)		
P	0.000		
Adjusted R square	0.443		
Constant	1.572 (−2.037 to 2.493)		
	O.R.	C.I. 95%	p
Lithium therapy	0.185	0–9.628	0.149
Age	1.005	0.76–1.146	0.944
Gender	0.415	0.008–3.64	0.407
Presence of psychotic symptoms	0.692	0.003–7.39	0.726
Aggressive behavior	0.130	0.003–5.236	0.103
Seasonality	1.172	0.002–4.764	0.870
Duration of illness	1.026	0.862–1.215	0.668
Lifetime number of affective episodes (1–10)	-	0.852–1.356	0.229
Lifetime number of affective episodes (11–21)	11.233	0.523–1.112	0.098
Lifetime number of affective episodes (>22)	12.099	0.654–1.288	0.139
Lifetime number of psychiatric admissions	0.702	0.123–1.789	0.598
brief TEMPS-M subscores			
Depressive	0.875	0.448–1.096	0.294
Hyperthymic	0.800	0.526–1021	0.018
Anxious	1.098	0.681–1.428	0.461
Cyclothymic	1.127	0.974–2.015	0.271
Irritable	1.064	0.719–1.147	0.414

F-test; df, degree of freedom; C.I., confidence interval; O.R., Odds Ratio.

4. Discussion

The impact of affective temperaments on the risk of suicidal behavior is an emerging theme in the field of mental health [18,37,38]. Our sample is mainly composed of BD-II patients, considered at the highest risk of suicide attempts among patients with the bipolar spectrum [39]. Recent research showed that suicide attempts are 1.5 times more frequent among women than men and that the risk of suicide attempts decreases from BDII to major depression, BDI, other psychiatric disorders and to psychotic disorders, which carry the lowest risk [40]. This can be explained by the evidence that BDII patients experience more chronicity [41], higher rates of rapid cycling [42], greater disabling depressive symptoms [39], a higher probability of misdiagnosis [41], more anxiety disorders in comorbidity [43], agitated depression and residual symptoms [44]. Our study confirms that hyperthymic temperament is associated with a reduced risk of suicide attempts in BD patients, while depressive, cyclothymic and anxious temperaments have a strong association with suicide attempts [45]. These findings are in line with previous reports [16,22,46]. Hyperthymic temperament may exert protective effects in different ways, such as better drive, greater energy, more ambition, as well as better coping and decrease the risk of suicidal behavior [19,46]. On the other hand, the low rating of hyperthymic temperament has been associated with increased hopelessness, an important predictor of suicide attempts [47]. Contrary to previous studies [28], our data do not confirm the role of irritable temperament on suicide risk, probably due to the small sample size. In our study emerged that psychotic symptoms are more represented in patients with a history of suicide attempts particularly during mixed episodes [45]. Several studies have suggested that individuals who experience psychotic symptoms have an increased sensitivity to stress, in terms of affective reactions to life events [48], as well as poorer coping skills [49], which may contribute to a greater risk of suicidal behavior when faced with acute life stressors. Other potential mechanisms may be the presence of shared risk factors for suicidal behavior and psychotic symptoms, including traumatic early life experiences, especially physical and sexual abuse [45], as reported by a recent meta-analysis by Ng et al. [50]. Therefore, mixed states, both with or without psychotic symptoms, are associated with an elevated risk of suicidal behavior, due to a greater proportion of time spent being depressed than patients without mixed episodes [51]. Furthermore, our study has outlined several clinical characteristics of violent suicide attempters. Rapid cycling patients were more likely to be violent attempters, as well as patients with BD-I and with cyclothymic temperament. Increased impulsivity, which is often a characteristic of cyclothymic temperament, is associated with a worse prognosis of BD [52,53], and with a more severe clinical course of the disease with history of rapid cycling, mixed episodes and substance abuse [54]. Our findings are in line with other studies showing that cyclothymic temperament is associated with a behavioral instability, increased sensitivity to a stressful event and higher levels of impulsivity [22,55–57], and a risk factor for suicide attempts [21]. Therefore, identifying those conditions such as cyclothymic temperament, a rapid cycling course or mixed episodes, more related to an impulsive dimension in patients with BD, could help to more easily typify a subpopulation of patients at risk of committing violent suicide attempts.

The higher rates of cyclothymic dominant temperament among patients with BD have been widely shown in several studies [38,57]. There is still an open debate whether cyclothymic temperaments and cyclothymia as a psychiatric disorder have overlapping characteristics. In particular, cyclothymia has been conceptualized as the extreme of a cyclothymic temperament, characterized by high rates of impulsivity, emotional lability and mood swings [55]; it is estimated that up to one third of patients with cyclothymia have more possibilities to develop BD, particularly the type II [58]. A great number of patients are misclassified as bipolar, depressed or with a personality disorder instead of receiving a diagnosis of cyclothymia by the use of DSM-5 diagnostic criteria [55,59,60]; thus, is it possible that patients with a diagnosis of cyclothymia with BDs have been included in the study. A broader approach, considering not only a categorical diagnosis based on strict DSM-5 criteria but including temperamental dimension also, could help to better identify patients with cyclothymia and plan individualized treatments [50].

Underdiagnosis or misdiagnosis are relatively common in BD [61,62], and they are linked with the presence of milder symptoms not fitting a BD diagnosis, but falling into the "soft bipolar spectrum" definition [63]. In particular, Akiskal and Pinto (1999) [63] described two subtypes of bipolar spectrum not associated with manic or hypomanic state: bipolar II1/2 (depression superimposed on cyclothymic temperament) and bipolar IV (depression superimposed on hyperthymic temperament). A recent work by Goto and colleagues [64] proved that depression in those who have cyclothymic (bipolar II1/2) and hyperthymic temperament (bipolar IV) may predict bipolarity, giving validity to the bipolar II 1/2 and bipolar IV concepts; this is in line with our results on cyclothymic temperament which is highly represented in the total sample and significantly higher in violent attempters.

It is important to emphasize that this was an exploratory study with several potential limitations. The small sample size reduces the statistical power of our findings, especially in the sub-analysis made in the population of violent suicide attempters. Furthermore, we could not assess some socio-demographic characteristics and levels of education. Moreover, we only collected data on lithium treatment, but we have no data on other psychiatric medications. The time during which the study was conducted was relatively short; this can affect, for example, data on seasonality. Finally, data on aggression, as well as on clinical course, number or duration of admissions, presence of psychotic symptoms, were not assessed with objective measures, but they were referred by patients. The paper has also several strengths, such as the naturalistic setting and the fact that it is one of the first clinical studies on the possible role of affective temperaments in patients with BD. Moreover, in this study we evaluated the subpopulation of violent suicide attempters of BD patients, which can be considered an early detection target and can be taken into account for personalized treatments for BD.

5. Conclusions

Our study outlined several clinical and temperamental characteristics of violent suicide attempters. Temperaments, in particular the affective ones, should be routinely assessed in clinical settings in order to identify people at higher risk of suicide attempts and to develop preventive programs, although it would be reductive to build a "suicide attempter profile" only on the basis of temperaments. A wider clinical evaluation, including also different clinical aspects such as current affective episodes and severity of the disease, pharmacological treatments, and the use of coping strategies in stressful situations should be taken into consideration in order to have effective early interventions.

Author Contributions: Conceptualization, A.F., M.L. and G.F. and Y.Y.; methodology, G.S., L.J.S., V.C., F.Z., M.C.; formal analysis, G.S., M.L. and G.F.; writing—original draft preparation, G.F., M.L., V.C., F.Z., M.C.; writing—review and editing, A.F., M.L., F.Z.; supervision, A.F.

Funding: This research received no external funding.

Conflicts of Interest: The authors declare no conflict of interest.

References

1. WHO. *Suicide Data*; WHO: Geneva, Switzerland, 2018.
2. Bachmann, S. Epidemiology of Suicide and the Psychiatric Perspective. *Int. J. Environ. Res. Public Health* **2018**, *15*, 1425. [CrossRef] [PubMed]
3. Gonda, X.; Pompili, M.; Serafini, G.; Montebovi, F.; Campi, S.; Dome, P.; Duleba, T.; Girardi, P.; Rihmer, Z. Suicidal behavior in bipolar disorder: Epidemiology, characteristics and major risk factors. *J. Affect. Disord.* **2012**, *143*, 16–26. [CrossRef] [PubMed]
4. Schaffer, A.; Isometsa, E.T.; Tondo, L.; H Moreno, D.; Turecki, G.; Reis, C.; Cassidy, F.; Sinyor, M.; Azorin, J.-M.; Kessing, L.V.; et al. International Society for Bipolar Disorders Task Force on Suicide: Meta-analyses and meta-regression of correlates of suicide attempts and suicide deaths in bipolar disorder. *Bipolar Disord.* **2015**, *17*, 1–16. [CrossRef] [PubMed]

5. Vijayakumar, L.; Phillips, M.R.; Silverman, M.M.; Gunnell, D.; Carli, V. Suicide. In *Mental, Neurological, and Substance Use Disorders: Disease Control Priorities*; Patel, V., Chisholm, D., Dua, T., Laxminarayan, R., Medina-Mora, M.E., Eds.; The International Bank for Reconstruction and Development/The World Bank: Washington, DC, USA, 2016; ISBN 9781464804267.
6. Runeson, B.; Tidemalm, D.; Dahlin, M.; Lichtenstein, P.; Langstrom, N. Method of attempted suicide as predictor of subsequent successful suicide: National long term cohort study. *BMJ* **2010**, *341*, c3222. [CrossRef] [PubMed]
7. Stenbacka, M.; Jokinen, J. Violent and non-violent methods of attempted and completed suicide in Swedish young men: The role of early risk factors. *BMC Psychiatry* **2015**, *15*, 196. [CrossRef]
8. Gunnell, D.; Bennewith, O.; Hawton, K.; Simkin, S.; Kapur, N. The epidemiology and prevention of suicide by hanging: A systematic review. *Int. J. Epidemiol.* **2005**, *34*, 433–442. [CrossRef]
9. Asberg, M.; Traskman, L.; Thoren, P. 5-HIAA in the cerebrospinal fluid. A biochemical suicide predictor? *Arch. Gen. Psychiatry* **1976**, *33*, 1193–1197. [CrossRef]
10. Giner, L.; Jaussent, I.; Olié, E.; Béziat, S.; Guillaume, S.; Baca-Garcia, E.; Lopez-Castroman, J.; Courtet, P. Violent and serious suicide attempters: One step closer to suicide? *J. Clin. Psychiatry* **2014**, *75*, e191–e197. [CrossRef]
11. Penas-Lledo, E.; Guillaume, S.; Delgado, A.; Naranjo, M.E.G.; Jaussent, I.; LLerena, A.; Courtet, P. ABCB1 gene polymorphisms and violent suicide attempt among survivors. *J. Psychiatry Res.* **2015**, *61*, 52–56. [CrossRef]
12. Dumais, A.; Lesage, A.D.; Lalovic, A.; Seguin, M.; Tousignant, M.; Chawky, N.; Turecki, G. Is violent method of suicide a behavioral marker of lifetime aggression? *Am. J. Psychiatry* **2005**, *162*, 1375–1378. [CrossRef]
13. Costa Lda, S.; Alencar, Á.P.; Nascimento Neto, P.J.; dos Santos Mdo, S.; da Silva, C.G.; Pinheiro Sde, F.; Silveira, R.T.; Bianco, B.A.; Pinheiro, R.F., Jr.; de Lima, M.A.; et al. Risk factors for suicide in bipolar disorder: A systematic review. *J. Affect. Disord.* **2015**, *170*, 237–254. [CrossRef]
14. Hansson, C.; Joas, E.; Palsson, E.; Hawton, K.; Runeson, B.; Landen, M. Risk factors for suicide in bipolar disorder: A cohort study of 12 850 patients. *Acta Psychiatr. Scand.* **2018**, *138*, 456–463. [CrossRef] [PubMed]
15. Perroud, N.; Baud, P.; Ardu, S.; Krejci, I.; Mouthon, D.; Vessaz, M.; Guillaume, S.; Jaussent, I.; Olie, E.; Malafosse, A.; et al. Temperament personality profiles in suicidal behaviour: An investigation of associated demographic, clinical and genetic factors. *J. Affect. Disord.* **2013**, *146*, 246–253. [CrossRef] [PubMed]
16. Rihmer, Z.; Akiskal, K.K.; Rihmer, A.; Akiskal, H.S. Current research on affective temperaments. *Curr. Opin. Psychiatry* **2010**, *23*, 12–18. [CrossRef] [PubMed]
17. Akiskal, H.S.; Akiskal, K. Cyclothymic, hyperthymic, and depressive temperaments as subaffective variants of mood disorders. In *Annual Review, Vol. II*; Tasman, A., Riba, M.B., Eds.; American Psychiatric Press: Washington, DC, USA, 1992; pp. 43–62.
18. Akiskal, H.S.; Akiskal, K.K.; Haykal, R.F.; Manning, J.S.; Connor, P.D. TEMPS-A: Progress towards validation of a self-rated clinical version of the Temperament Evaluation of the Memphis, Pisa, Paris, and San Diego Autoquestionnaire. *J. Affect. Disord.* **2005**, *85*, 3–16. [CrossRef] [PubMed]
19. Pompili, M.; Innamorati, M.; Gonda, X.; Serafini, G.; Sarno, S.; Erbuto, D.; Palermo, M.; Elena Seretti, M.; Stefani, H.; Lester, D.; et al. Affective temperaments and hopelessness as predictors of health and social functioning in mood disorder patients: A prospective follow-up study. *J. Affect. Disord.* **2013**, *150*, 216–222. [CrossRef]
20. Tondo, L.; Vazquez, G.H.; Sani, G.; Pinna, M.; Baldessarini, R.J. Association of suicidal risk with ratings of affective temperaments. *J. Affect. Disord.* **2018**, *229*, 322–327. [CrossRef] [PubMed]
21. Baldessarini, R.J.; Vazquez, G.H.; Tondo, L. Affective temperaments and suicidal ideation and behavior in mood and anxiety disorder patients. *J. Affect. Disord.* **2016**, *198*, 78–82. [CrossRef]
22. Pompili, M.; Rihmer, Z.; Akiskal, H.S.; Innamorati, M.; Iliceto, P.; Akiskal, K.K.; Lester, D.; Narciso, V.; Ferracuti, S.; Tatarelli, R.; et al. Temperament and personality dimensions in suicidal and nonsuicidal psychiatric inpatients. *Psychopathology* **2008**, *41*, 313–321. [CrossRef]
23. Rihmer, A.; Rozsa, S.; Rihmer, Z.; Gonda, X.; Akiskal, K.K.; Akiskal, H.S. Affective temperaments, as measured by TEMPS-A, among nonviolent suicide attempters. *J. Affect. Disord.* **2009**, *116*, 18–22. [CrossRef]
24. Dolenc, B.; Dernovšek, M.Z.; Sprah, L.; Tavcar, R.; Perugi, G.; Akiskal, H.S. Relationship between affective temperaments and aggression in euthymic patients with bipolar mood disorder and major depressive disorder. *J. Affect. Disord.* **2015**, *174*, 13–18. [CrossRef] [PubMed]

25. Walsh, M.A.; Royal, A.M.; Barrantes-Vidal, N.; Kwapil, T.R. The association of affective temperaments with impairment and psychopathology in a young adult sample. *J. Affect. Disord.* **2012**, *141*, 373–381. [CrossRef] [PubMed]
26. Akiskal, H.S.; Placidi, G.F.; Maremmani, I.; Signoretta, S.; Liguori, A.; Gervasi, R.; Mallya, G.; Puzantian, V.R. TEMPS-I: Delineating the most discriminant traits of the cyclothymic, depressive, hyperthymic and irritable temperaments in a nonpatient population. *J. Affect. Disord.* **1998**, *51*, 7–19. [CrossRef]
27. Elias, L.R.; Kohler, C.A.; Stubbs, B.; Maciel, B.R.; Cavalcante, L.M.; Vale, A.M.O.; Gonda, X.; Quevedo, J.; Hyphantis, T.N.; Soares, J.C.; et al. Measuring affective temperaments: A systematic review of validation studies of the Temperament Evaluation in Memphis Pisa and San Diego (TEMPS) instruments. *J. Affect. Disord.* **2017**, *212*, 25–37. [CrossRef]
28. Vazquez, G.H.; Gonda, X.; Lolich, M.; Tondo, L.; Baldessarini, R.J. Suicidal Risk and Affective Temperaments, Evaluated with the TEMPS-A Scale: A Systematic Review. *Harv. Rev. Psychiatry* **2018**, *26*, 8–18. [CrossRef] [PubMed]
29. Nivoli, A.M.A.; Pacchiarotti, I.; Rosa, A.R.; Popovic, D.; Murru, A.; Valenti, M.; Bonnin, C.M.; Grande, I.; Sanchez-Moreno, J.; Vieta, E.; et al. Gender differences in a cohort study of 604 bipolar patients: The role of predominant polarity. *J. Affect. Disord.* **2011**, *133*, 443–449. [CrossRef]
30. Neves, F.S.; Malloy-Diniz, L.F.; Correa, H. Suicidal behavior in bipolar disorder: What is the influence of psychiatric comorbidities? *J. Clin. Psychiatry* **2009**, *70*, 13–18. [CrossRef]
31. Gonda, X.; Fountoulakis, K.N.; Harro, J.; Pompili, M.; Akiskal, H.S.; Bagdy, G.; Rihmer, Z. The possible contributory role of the S allele of 5-HTTLPR in the emergence of suicidality. *J. Psychopharmacol.* **2011**, *25*, 857–866. [CrossRef]
32. Erfurth, A.; Gerlach, A.L.; Hellweg, I.; Boenigk, I.; Michael, N.; Akiskal, H.S. Studies on a German (Munster) version of the temperament auto-questionnaire TEMPS-A: Construction and validation of the briefTEMPS-M. *J. Affect. Disord.* **2005**, *85*, 53–69. [CrossRef]
33. Naderer, A.; Keller, F.; Plener, P.; Unseld, M.; Lesch, O.M.; Walter, H.; Erfurth, A.; Kapusta, N.D. The brief TEMPS-M temperament questionnaire: A psychometric evaluation in an Austrian sample. *J. Affect. Disord.* **2015**, *188*, 43–46. [CrossRef]
34. Fico, G.; Luciano, M.; Sampogna, G.; Zinno, F.; Steardo, L., Jr.; Perugi, G.; Pompili, M.; Tortorella, A.; Volpe, U.; Fiorillo, A.; et al. Validation of the brief TEMPS-M temperament questionnaire in a clinical Italian sample of bipolar and cyclothymic patients. *J. Affect. Disord* **2019**, in press.
35. Tor, E.N.; Cloninger, R.; Przybeck, T.R.; Svrakic, D.; Wetzel, R.D. *TCI-Guide to Its Development and Use*; Center for Psychobiology of Personality Washington University: St. Louis, MO, USA, 2014.
36. Fossati, A.; Cloninger, C.R.; Villa, D.; Borroni, S.; Grazioli, F.; Giarolli, L.; Battaglia, M.; Maffei, C. Reliability and validity of the Italian version of the Temperament and Character Inventory-Revised in an outpatient sample. *Compr. Psychiatry* **2007**, *48*, 380–387. [CrossRef] [PubMed]
37. Karam, E.G.; Salamoun, M.M.; Yeretzian, J.S.; Mneimneh, Z.N.; Karam, A.N.; Fayyad, J.; Hantouche, E.; Akiskal, K.; Akiskal, H.S. The role of anxious and hyperthymic temperaments in mental disorders: A national epidemiologic study. *World Psychiatry* **2010**, *9*, 103–110. [CrossRef] [PubMed]
38. Kochman, F.J.; Hantouche, E.G.; Ferrari, P.; Lancrenon, S.; Bayart, D.; Akiskal, H.S. Cyclothymic temperament as a prospective predictor of bipolarity and suicidality in children and adolescents with major depressive disorder. *J. Affect. Disord.* **2005**, *85*, 181–189. [CrossRef] [PubMed]
39. Rihmer, Z.; Kiss, K. Bipolar disorders and suicidal behaviour. *Bipolar Disord.* **2002**, *4*, 21–25. [CrossRef] [PubMed]
40. Pompili, M.; Baldessarini, R.J.; Innamorati, M.; Vazquez, G.H.; Rihmer, Z.; Gonda, X.; Forte, A.; Lamis, D.A.; Erbuto, D.; Serafini, G.; et al. Temperaments in psychotic and major affective disorders. *J. Affect. Disord.* **2018**, *225*, 195–200. [CrossRef] [PubMed]
41. Vieta, E.; Benabarre, A.; Colom, F.; Gasto, C.; Nieto, E.; Otero, A.; Vallejo, J. Suicidal behavior in bipolar I and bipolar II disorder. *J. Nerv. Ment. Dis.* **1997**, *185*, 407–409. [CrossRef] [PubMed]
42. Maj, M.; Pirozzi, R.; Formicola, A.M.; Tortorella, A. Reliability and validity of four alternative definitions of rapid-cycling bipolar disorder. *Am. J. Psychiatry* **1999**, *156*, 1421–1424.
43. Henry, C.; Van den Bulke, D.; Bellivier, F.; Etain, B.; Rouillon, F.; Leboyer, M. Anxiety disorders in 318 bipolar patients: Prevalence and impact on illness severity and response to mood stabilizer. *J. Clin. Psychiatry* **2003**, *64*, 331–335. [CrossRef]

44. Benazzi, F. Prevalence and clinical correlates of residual depressive symptoms in bipolar II disorder. *Psychother. Psychosom.* **2001**, *70*, 232–238. [CrossRef]
45. Kelleher, I.; Corcoran, P.; Keeley, H.; Wigman, J.T.W.; Devlin, N.; Ramsay, H.; Wasserman, C.; Carli, V.; Sarchiapone, M.; Hoven, C.; et al. Psychotic symptoms and population risk for suicide attempt: A prospective cohort study. *JAMA Psychiatry* **2013**, *70*, 940–948. [CrossRef] [PubMed]
46. Vazquez, G.H.; Gonda, X.; Zaratiegui, R.; Lorenzo, L.S.; Akiskal, K.; Akiskal, H.S. Hyperthymic temperament may protect against suicidal ideation. *J. Affect. Disord.* **2010**, *127*, 38–42. [CrossRef] [PubMed]
47. Gonda, X.; Fountoulakis, K.N.; Kaprinis, G.; Rihmer, Z. Prediction and prevention of suicide in patients with unipolar depression and anxiety. *Ann. Gen. Psychiatry* **2007**, *6*, 23. [CrossRef] [PubMed]
48. Lataster, T.; Wichers, M.; Jacobs, N.; Mengelers, R.; Derom, C.; Thiery, E.; Van Os, J.; Myin-Germeys, I. Does reactivity to stress cosegregate with subclinical psychosis? A general population twin study. *Acta Psychiatr. Scand.* **2009**, *119*, 45–53. [CrossRef] [PubMed]
49. Wigman, J.T.W.; Devlin, N.; Kelleher, I.; Murtagh, A.; Harley, M.; Kehoe, A.; Fitzpatrick, C.; Cannon, M. Psychotic symptoms, functioning and coping in adolescents with mental illness. *BMC Psychiatry* **2014**, *14*, 97. [CrossRef] [PubMed]
50. Perugi, G.; Hantouche, E.; Vannucchi, G. Diagnosis and Treatment of Cyclothymia: The "Primacy" of Temperament. *Curr. Neuropharmacol.* **2017**, *15*, 372–379. [CrossRef] [PubMed]
51. Persons, J.E.; Coryell, W.H.; Solomon, D.A.; Keller, M.B.; Endicott, J.; Fiedorowicz, J.G. Mixed state and suicide: Is the effect of mixed state on suicidal behavior more than the sum of its parts? *Bipolar Disord.* **2018**, *20*, 35–41. [CrossRef]
52. Moeller, F.G.; Barratt, E.S.; Dougherty, D.M.; Schmitz, J.M.; Swann, A.C. Psychiatric aspects of impulsivity. *Am. J. Psychiatry* **2001**, *158*, 1783–1793. [CrossRef]
53. Swann, A.C.; Anderson, J.C.; Dougherty, D.M.; Moeller, F.G. Measurement of inter-episode impulsivity in bipolar disorder. *Psychiatry Res.* **2001**, *101*, 195–197. [CrossRef]
54. Etain, B.; Mathieu, F.; Liquet, S.; Raust, A.; Cochet, B.; Richard, J.R.; Gard, S.; Zanouy, L.; Kahn, J.P.; Cohen, R.F.; et al. Clinical features associated with trait-impulsiveness in euthymic bipolar disorder patients. *J. Affect. Disord.* **2013**, *144*, 240–247. [CrossRef]
55. Perugi, G.; Hantouche, E.; Vannucchi, G.; Pinto, O. Cyclothymia reloaded: A reappraisal of the most misconceived affective disorder. *J. Affect. Disord.* **2015**, *183*, 119–133. [CrossRef] [PubMed]
56. Popovic, D.; Vieta, E.; Azorin, J.-M.; Angst, J.; Bowden, C.L.; Mosolov, S.; Young, A.H.; Perugi, G. Suicide attempts in major depressive episode: Evidence from the BRIDGE-II-Mix study. *Bipolar Disord.* **2015**, *17*, 795–803. [CrossRef] [PubMed]
57. Jiménez, E.; Bonnín, C.D.M.; Solé, B.; Sánchez-Moreno, J.; Reinares, M.; Torrent, C.; Torres, I.; Salagre, E.; Varo, C.; Ruíz, V.; et al. Spanish validation of the Barcelona TEMPS-A questionnaire in patients with bipolar disorder and general population. *J. Affect. Disord.* **2019**, *249*, 199–207. [CrossRef] [PubMed]
58. Vieta, E.; Berk, M.; Schulze, T.G.; Carvalho, A.F.; Suppes, T.; Calabrese, J.R.; Gao, K.; Miskowiak, K.W.; Grande, I. Bipolar disorders. *Nat. Rev. Dis. Prim.* **2018**, *4*, 18008. [CrossRef] [PubMed]
59. Utsumi, T.; Sasaki, T.; Shimada, I.; Mabuchi, M.; Motonaga, T.; Ohtani, T.; Tochigi, M.; Kato, N.; Nanko, S. Clinical features of soft bipolarity in major depressive inpatients. *Psychiatry Clin. Neurosci.* **2006**, *60*, 611–615. [CrossRef]
60. Perugi, G.; Toni, C.; Travierso, M.C.; Akiskal, H.S. The role of cyclothymia in atypical depression: Toward a data-based reconceptualization of the borderline-bipolar II connection. *J. Affect. Disord.* **2003**, *73*, 87–98. [CrossRef]
61. Katzow, J.J.; Hsu, D.J.; Ghaemi, S.N. The bipolar spectrum: A clinical perspective. *Bipolar Disord.* **2003**, *5*, 436–442. [CrossRef]
62. De Fruyt, J.; Demyttenaere, K. Bipolar (spectrum) disorder and mood stabilization: Standing at the crossroads? *Psychother. Psychosom.* **2007**, *76*, 77–88. [CrossRef]

63. Akiskal, H.S.; Pinto, O. The evolving bipolar spectrum. Prototypes, I., II, III, and IV. *Psychiatr. Clin. N. Am.* **1999**, *22*, 517–534. [CrossRef]
64. Goto, S.; Terao, T.; Hoaki, N.; Wang, Y. Cyclothymic and hyperthymic temperaments may predict bipolarity in major depressive disorder: A supportive evidence for bipolar II1/2 and IV. *J. Affect. Disord.* **2011**, *129*, 34–38. [CrossRef]

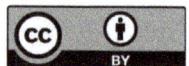

© 2019 by the authors. Licensee MDPI, Basel, Switzerland. This article is an open access article distributed under the terms and conditions of the Creative Commons Attribution (CC BY) license (http://creativecommons.org/licenses/by/4.0/).

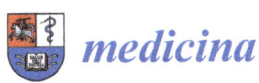

Review

Cytomegalovirus Seropositivity and Suicidal Behavior: A Mini-Review

Marco Paolini [1], David Lester [2], Michael Hawkins [3], Ameth Hawkins-Villarreal [4,5,†], Denise Erbuto [6], Andrea Fiorillo [7] and Maurizio Pompili [6,*]

1. Psychiatry Residency Training Program, Faculty of Medicine and Psychology, Sapienza University of Rome, 00185 Rome, Italy; marcopao88@gmail.com
2. Psychology Program, Stockton University, Galloway, NJ 08205, USA; David.Lester@stockton.edu
3. Department of Psychiatry, University of Toronto, Toronto, ON M5S, Canada; mhawkins@shn.ca
4. Fetal Medicine Research Center, BCNatal-Barcelona Center for Maternal-Fetal and Neonatal Medicine, University of Barcelona, 08028 Barcelona, Spain; amethhawk@gmail.com
5. Fetal Medicine Service, Obstetrics Department, "Saint Thomas" Hospital, University of Panama, Panama City 0843, Panama
6. Department of Neurosciences, Mental Health and Sensory Organs, Suicide Prevention Center, Sant'Andrea Hospital, Sapienza University of Rome, 00185 Rome, Italy; denise.erbuto@gmail.com
7. Department of Psychiatry, University of Campania Luigi Vanvitelli, 80138 Naples, Italy; andrea.fiorillo@unicampania.it
* Correspondence: maurizio.pompili@uniroma1.it
† On behalf of the Iberoamerican Research Network in Translational, Molecular and Maternal Fetal Medicine.

Received: 6 October 2019; Accepted: 9 December 2019; Published: 12 December 2019

Abstract: *Background and objectives*: In recent years, a growing body of research has focused on identifying possible biological markers for suicidal behavior, including infective and immunological markers. In this paper, our aim was to review available evidence concerning the association between cytomegalovirus (CMV) infection and suicide. *Materials and Methods*: A systematic search according to the PRISMA statement was performed on Pubmed. After the screening procedure, we identified five relevant papers. *Results*: We found inconsistent evidence linking CMV infection and suicide, with some papers reporting an association between CMV seropositivity and suicidal behavior, and others not finding the association. *Conclusions*: With the evidence available presently, it is not possible to infer whether there is a correlation between suicide and CMV infection.

Keywords: suicide; CMV; cytomegalovirus; biomarker; antibodies; review

1. Introduction

Although suicide research has made many advances [1], suicide remains an unpredictable [2] but leading cause of death. There are many known indicators/risk factors that can alert physicians' of those at risk of suicide, including clinical (e.g., psychiatric illness, substance use, previous attempts, medical illness), demographic (e.g., male sex, older age, living alone), genetic, and psychological (e.g., unemployment, interpersonal conflict) factors.

As research advances, many have wondered whether there are biological markers that could help clinicians in the assessment and management of individuals at risk of suicide [3]. In recent years, viral infections have received closer attention as a possible target in suicide research. Among these, cytomegalovirus (CMV) infection has been associated with the development of psychiatric disorders (e.g., schizophrenia and mood disorders) [4–8], neurodevelopmental disorders (e.g., autism) [9,10], neurocognitive disorders (e.g., Alzheimer's disease) [11], and suicide attempts and completions [12–14].

Cytomegalovirus (CMV) prevalence varies by population, with an estimated 40% to 100% of individuals infected [15,16]. Seroprevalence tends to be high in lower socio-economic groups and ethnic minority populations. Because of the high seroprevalence, a large reservoir of CMV continuously exists in the population [17]. CMV remains a major cause of congenital infection and disease during pregnancy around the world. In particular, congenital infection with human cytomegalovirus (HCMV) is a major cause of fetal brain damage [18–20]. CMV has a specific neurotropism that is evident from its predominance in central nervous system (CNS) abnormalities observed in symptomatic congenital infection (sensorineural hearing loss, neurological impairments and neurodevelopmental delay [21–24]).

In children and adults, both primary cytomegalovirus infection and reactivations are typically asymptomatic and, as a result, many people are unaware that they have been infected. The infection can lead, however, to an inflammatory response in the brain both in immune-compromised and immune-competent patients [25–27]. Recently, it has been suggested that neuroinflammation and activated microglia play an important role in the pathogenesis of suicide and suicidal behavior [28–30].

The aim of the present paper was to review all available evidence regarding CMV seropositivity and suicidal behavior.

2. Materials and Methods

For this review, we followed a systematic procedure in order to identify all peer-reviewed studies concerning CMV seropositivity and suicide. First, we performed a bibliographic search on Pubmed on 14 May 2019, using the following keywords: "(CMV OR cytomegalovirus or herpesvir*) AND (suicid* OR "self-harm" OR "self-killing")". We then searched for additional relevant papers after reviewing the works cited in the papers identified, and through the "relevant articles" section on Pubmed. This search resulted in 409 papers. We then applied our inclusion and exclusion criteria. The selection procedure was carried out according to the PRISMA statement (see Figure 1).

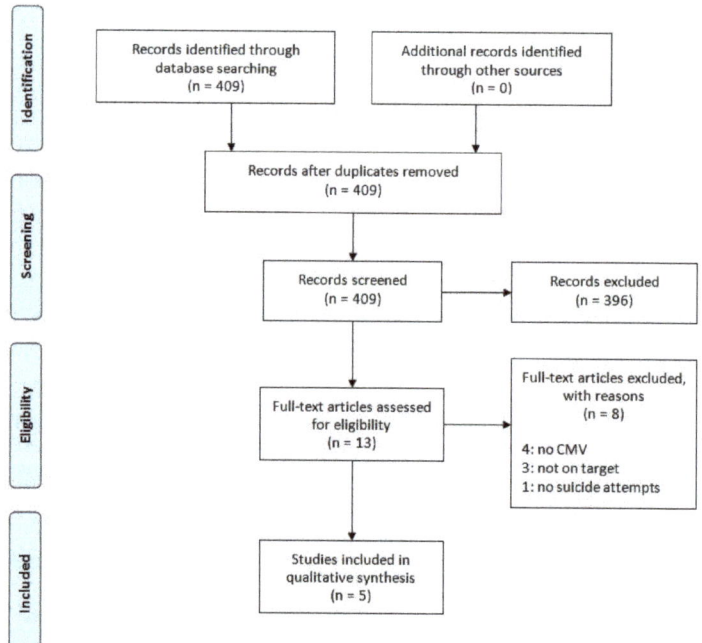

Figure 1. PRISMA flow diagram.

In order to be included, papers had to fulfil the following criterion—namely serological studies of anti-CMV antibodies in patients with previous or current suicide attempt(s) versus controls. Our exclusion criteria were: the absence of a control group, the absence of suicidal behaviour in the subjects, and post-mortem studies.

3. Results

Of the original 409 papers found, five articles met both the inclusion and exclusion criteria (see Figure 1). Two of these studies were performed on or had a control group drawn from the general population [12,31]; the other three only concerned people with serious mental illness [13,14,32].

3.1. Studies in Healthy Subjects

In the first group of papers, an association between CMV seropositivity and attempted suicide was reported (see Table 1). In a case-control study of 12,500 people, Burgdorf et al. [12] studied blood donors from the Danish Blood Donor Study [33], of whom 655 had attempted or completed suicide by the time of the study, 2591 had a psychiatric diagnosis, and 2724 had been in a traffic accidents. These individuals were compared to blood donors without these behaviours or a psychiatric diagnosis matched for age and sex. Burgordorf et al. found that 60.8% of the sample was infected with CMV [12]. The presence of CMV was associated with having any psychiatric diagnosis (OR = 1.17). In the blood donors who exhibited suicidal behaviour (i.e., those with at least one suicide attempt either before or after the blood donation and those who completed suicide after the blood donation), there was a higher prevalence of anti-CMV IgG compared to the controls (OR 1.31, 95% CI 1.10–1.56). However, for people who had attempted or died from suicide only after the blood donation (a nested case control study performed in order to account for temporality and to consider only cases in which the exposure precedes the outcome), CMV infection was no longer associated with these behaviors (OR = 1.18, 95% CI 0.50–2.82). As noted in the paper itself, a possible explanation for this discrepancy could be the small number of individuals having committed or attempted suicide after the blood collection [12].

Zhang et al. (2012) [31], in a cross-sectional observational study on a much smaller sample, compared 54 people who had attempted suicide with 30 controls. No statistically significant association between CMV seropositivity and suicidal behavior was found, although a slightly higher prevalence of anti-CMV IgG was found in people who had attempted suicide compared to the controls (33/53, 62.2% vs. 16/29, 55.1%).

3.2. Studies in Psychiatric Patients

Studies performed on people with serious mental illness reported more mixed results (see Table 2). Dickerson et al. [13], in a prospective study, followed 733 patients with schizophrenia spectrum disorders, 483 patients with bipolar disorder and 76 patients with major depressive disorder for an average of 8.15 years. Those who died by suicide ($n = 16$) had significantly higher levels of anti-CMV IgG. Death from suicide was also associated with higher levels of IgG antibodies after adjusting for demographics, psychiatric diagnosis, and psychiatric symptom severity. Suicide risk ranged from 2.51 (95% CI = 0.89–7.10, $p < 0.082$) for individuals with levels greater than or equal to 1 (the cut-off value) to 6.45 (95% CI = 2.15–19.32, $p = 0.001$) for individuals with levels ≥ 3 times the cut-off value. In a multiple regression analysis, male sex, being Caucasian, being separated/divorced and CMV IgG antibody levels predicted suicide.

Table 1. Studies in Healthy Subjects.

Study (Year)	Type of Study	Study Population	Case Population	Control Population	Analysis Method	Outcome
Burgdorf et al. [12]	Case control study	Data from 81,912 individuals from the Danish blood donor study. Total sample: 11,546 cases and controls	Blood donors who died by suicide or engaged in suicide attempts ($n = 655$)	Blood donors who did not die by suicide or engage in suicide attempts ($n = 6503$)	IgG anti cytomegalovirus (CMV). Solid phase ELISA	Seropositivity: 439/655 (67%) vs. 3886/6503 (59.7%), OR 1.31, 95% CI 1.10–1.56
Zhang et al. [31]	Cross-sectional observational study	Suicide attempters from inpatients at Lund University Hospital, Sweden. Controls from municipal population of Lund, Sweden. Total sample: 84 cases and controls	Patients admitted for suicide attempt ($n = 54$)	People randomly selected from the municipal population with no psychiatric condition or previous suicide attempt ($n = 30$)	IgG anti CMV, CMV titer. ELISA	Seropositivity: 33/53 (62.2%) vs. 16/29 (55.1%). CMV IgG titer: 99.5 (±86.9) vs. 91.3 (±92.0)

Table 2. Studies in Psychiatric Patient.

Study (Year)	Type of Study	Study Population	Case Population	Control Population	Analysis Method	Outcome
Dickerson et al. 2018 [13]	Prospective study with 16y FU	Individuals with previous diagnosis of schizophrenia spectrum disorder, bipolar disorder or major depressive disorder. Total sample: 1292 individuals	Individuals with serious mental illness who died by suicide ($n = 16$)	Individuals with serious mental illness who did not die by suicide ($n = 1276$)	IgG anti-CMV titer. Solid phase ELISA. Antibody levels expressed as a ratio between the test sample divided by that of a standard control sample.	CMV IgG titer: 3.35 (± 3.07) vs. 1.59 (± 1.90). Association found between increasing levels of antibodies and Hazard Ratios.
Dickerson et al. 2017 [14]	Cross-sectional study	Individuals with previous diagnosis of schizophrenia spectrum disorder, bipolar disorder or major depressive disorder. Total sample: 162 patients	Individuals with serious mental illness with previous suicide attempts ($n = 72$)	Individuals with serious mental illness without a previous suicide attempt ($n = 90$)	Anti-CMV IgG and IgM titer. Solid phase ELISA.	Association between suicide attempts and IgM anti CMV measured as a continuous variable (coefficient 0.151). Increased odds of suicide for levels of IgM anti CMV ≥ 75th and 90th percentiles (OR 3.02 and 6.31 respectively). No association with IgG.
Okusaga et al. 2011 [32]	Cross-sectional study	Patients diagnosed with schizophrenia through SCID, recruited in the Munich area of Germany. Total sample: 950 patients	351 individuals with schizophrenia with previous suicide attempts.	599 individuals with schizophrenia with no previous suicide attempt.	IgG anti-CMV. Solid phase ELISA.	Seropositivity for CMV not associated with a history of suicide attempt. No further data provided.

Dickerson, et al. [14] studied 162 patients with a psychiatric illness including patients with schizophrenia [n = 65], bipolar disorder [n = 59], and major depression [n = 38]. In the total sample, 72 (44%) had a history of attempted suicide. Those who attempted suicide had higher levels of CMV IgM antibodies, and the association was stronger with increasing levels of IgM antibodies (≥75th percentile OR = 3.02, 95% CI 1.08–8.44; ≥90th percentile OR = 6.31, 95% CI 1.17–33.9. $p = 0.032$). No association with IgG class antibodies was reported.

Okusaga et al. [32] studied 950 patients with a diagnosis of schizophrenia, of whom 351 (37%) had a history of attempted suicide. Seropositivity for CMV was not significantly associated with a history of suicide attempt.

4. Discussion

The evidence linking CMV seropositivity and suicide is limited. Our bibliographic search resulted in only five papers. Among these, one (Burgdorf et al. [12]) had a much larger sample size than the other four. Furthermore, the identified studies were methodologically heterogeneous, with some comparing CMV seropositivity between those who attempted or completed suicide with healthy controls, and others focused only on people with serious mental illnesses.

When compared to healthy controls, people with a history of suicide attempt(s) seem to have a higher prevalence of anti-CMV IgG, but the effect size seems to be small (Table 1 [12,31]). However, correlation does not imply causality, and, presently, it is not possible to say whether CMV infection is a risk factor for suicide. It may very well be that people with a higher suicide risk are also at a higher risk of contracting CMV infection. In this regard, Okusaga et al. [32] suggested that individuals with suicidal tendencies might engage in activities that increase the risk of exposure to infections—such as not washing vegetables thoroughly or eating undercooked meat.

In regards to people with severe mental illness, the results appear to be mixed. One study reported higher CMV IgG levels in patients with a mental illness (namely schizophrenia, bipolar disorder, and major depression) who died from suicide compared to controls [13], while another study found higher levels of IgM-class antibodies in those who had attempted suicide, but no difference concerning IgG [14]. A third study, carried out only on schizophrenic patients found no association [32].

This heterogeneity of findings could be partially explained by the fact that these studies involved patients with different psychiatric disorders (namely schizophrenia, bipolar disorder, and major depression). People with schizophrenia and psychotic spectrum disorders could have distinct features and a different pathophysiology leading to suicide compared to people with non-psychotic illnesses [34,35]. Other factors that may explain the reported differences between the studies examining the association between CMV infection and suicide is that these studies did not distinguish between acute CMV infection, chronic infection (either congenitally acquired or acquired as an adult), and reactivations of CMV infection. Dickerson et al. [14] suggested that the differences among the studies—in terms of immunoglobulin class—specificity may be related to methodological issues such as the format of the assay and the specificity of the immunoreagents. However, Dickerson et al. did not find that the elevated IgM levels encountered in their study were due to unspecific markers of infection, including naturally occurring antibodies or elevated IgM levels from reactivation from rheumatoid factors.

Previous studies have suggested an association between inflammation and increased suicide risk in people with a psychiatric illness [36], but whether the association between CMV infection and suicide exists is uncertain. Previous research in this area has found increased levels of inflammatory markers (e.g., interleukin-6) in patients with suicidal ideation and behaviour [37,38]. Activated interleukine-6 has been implicated also in acute fetal brain responses and long-term changes in brain development and behavior [39].

Much has been discussed about the effects of CMV infection on the brain of the fetus, but less is known about the effects of this infection on the adult brain, or the degree of brain damage in those with asymptomatic CMV infection. Congenital brain CMV infection is thought to be irreversible.

CMV affects many of the brain cells including microglia [40]. Microglial density has been found to be increased in people who have died from suicide. In contrast, no changes in microglial density have been observed between people with a psychiatric illness and healthy controls [41]. Either way, it is too soon to draw conclusions about the potential association between CMV infection and suicide. More studies are needed before causality can be implied.

To our knowledge, this is the first review concerning CMV seropositivity and suicide. The major limitation of this review is that our bibliographic search was conducted using only one database (Pubmed). Another limitation is that our search only resulted in five papers that were methodologically heterogeneous, thus rendering a meta-analytic procedure impossible.

5. Conclusions

The evidence linking CMV infection and suicide risk is scarce. To test this association further, studies comparing CMV seropositivity among psychotic and non-psychotic suicide attempters are needed.

Author Contributions: Conceptualization, M.P. (Marco Paolini) and M.P. (Maurizio Pompili); methodology, A.F.; investigation, D.E.; writing—original draft preparation, M.P. (Marco Paolini) and M.P. (Maurizio Pompili); writing—review and editing, D.L., M.H., A.H.-V.; supervision, M.P. (Marco Paolini) and M.P. (Maurizio Pompili).

Funding: This research received no external funding.

Conflicts of Interest: The authors declare no conflict of interest.

References

1. Niculescu, A.B.; Le-Niculescu, H.; Levey, D.F.; Phalen, P.L.; Dainton, H.L.; Roseberry, K.; Niculescu, E.M.; Niezer, J.O.; Williams, A.; Graham, D.L.; et al. Precision medicine for suicidality: From universality to subtypes and personalization. *Mol. Psychiatry* **2017**, *22*, 1250. [CrossRef] [PubMed]
2. Belsher, B.E.; Smolenski, D.J.; Pruitt, L.D.; Bush, N.E.; Beech, E.H.; Workman, D.E.; Morgan, R.L.; Evatt, D.P.; Tucker, J.; Skopp, N.A. Prediction Models for Suicide Attempts and Deaths: A Systematic Review and Simulation. *JAMA Psychiatry* **2019**, *76*, 642–651. [CrossRef] [PubMed]
3. Oquendo, M.A.; Sullivan, G.M.; Sudol, K.; Baca-Garcia, E.; Stanley, B.H.; Sublette, M.E.; Mann, J.J. Toward a biosignature for suicide. *Am. J. Psychiatry* **2014**, *171*, 1259–1277. [CrossRef] [PubMed]
4. Leweke, F.M.; Gerth, C.W.; Koethe, D.; Klosterkötter, J.; Ruslanova, I.; Krivogorsky, B.; Torrey, E.F.; Yolken, R.H. Antibodies to infectious agents in individuals with recent onset schizophrenia. *Eur. Arch. Psychiatr. Clin. Neurosci.* **2004**, *254*, 4–8. [CrossRef] [PubMed]
5. Mohagheghi, M.; Eftekharian, M.M.; Taheri, M.; Alikhani, M.Y. Determining the IgM and IgG antibodies titer against HSV1, HSV2 and CMV in the serum of schizophrenia patients. *Hum. Antibodies* **2018**, *26*, 87–93. [CrossRef] [PubMed]
6. Tedla, Y.; Shibre, T.; Ali, O.; Tadele, G.; Woldeamanuel, Y.; Asrat, D.; Aseffa, A.; Mihret, W.; Abebe, M.; Alem, A.; et al. Serum antibodies to Toxoplasma gondii and Herpesvidae family viruses in individuals with schizophrenia and bipolar disorder: A case-control study. *Ethiop. Med. J.* **2011**, *49*, 211–220.
7. Tanaka, T.; Matsuda, T.; Hayes, L.N.; Yang, S.; Rodriguez, K.; Severance, E.G.; Yolken, R.H.; Sawa, A.; Eaton, W.W. Infection and inflammation in schizophrenia and bipolar disorder. *Neurosci. Res.* **2017**, *115*, 59–63. [CrossRef]
8. Prossin, A.R.; Yolken, R.H.; Kamali, M.; Heitzeg, M.M.; Kaplow, J.B.; Coryell, W.H.; McInnis, M.G. Cytomegalovirus Antibody Elevation in Bipolar Disorder: Relation to Elevated Mood States. *Neural Plast.* **2015**, *2015*, 939780. [CrossRef]
9. Sweeten, T.L.; Posey, D.J.; McDougle, C.J. Brief report: Autistic disorder in three children with cytomegalovirus infection. *J. Autism Dev. Disord.* **2004**, *34*, 583–586. [CrossRef]
10. Garofoli, F.; Lombardi, G.; Orcesi, S.; Pisoni, C.; Mazzucchelli, I.; Angelini, M.; Balottin, U.; Stronati, M. An Italian Prospective Experience on the Association Between Congenital Cytomegalovirus Infection and Autistic Spectrum Disorder. *J. Autism Dev. Disord.* **2017**, *47*, 1490–1495. [CrossRef]

11. Sochocka, M.; Zwolińska, K.; Leszek, J. The Infectious Etiology of Alzheimer's Disease. *Curr. Neuropharmacol.* **2017**, *15*, 996–1009. [CrossRef] [PubMed]
12. Burgdorf, K.S.; Trabjerg, B.B.; Pedersen, M.G.; Nissen, J.; Banasik, K.; Pedersen, O.B.; Sørensen, E.; Nielsen, K.R.; Larsen, M.H.; Erikstrup, C.; et al. Large-scale study of Toxoplasma and Cytomegalovirus shows an association between infection and serious psychiatric disorders. *Brain Behav. Immun.* **2019**. [CrossRef] [PubMed]
13. Dickerson, F.; Origoni, A.; Schweinfurth, L.A.B.; Stallings, C.; Savage, C.L.G.; Sweeney, K.; Katsafanas, E.; Wilcox, H.C.; Khushalani, S.; Yolken, R. Clinical and Serological Predictors of Suicide in Schizophrenia and Major Mood Disorders. *J. Nerv. Ment. Dis.* **2018**, *206*, 173–178. [CrossRef] [PubMed]
14. Dickerson, F.; Wilcox, H.C.; Adamos, M.; Katsafanas, E.; Khushalani, S.; Origoni, A.; Savage, C.; Schweinfurth, L.; Stallings, C.; Sweeney, K.; et al. Suicide Attempts and Markers of Immune Response in Individuals with Serious Mental Illness. *J. Psychiatr. Res.* **2017**. [CrossRef] [PubMed]
15. Bate, S.L.; Dollard, S.C.; Cannon, M.J. Cytomegalovirus seroprevalence in the United States: The national health and nutrition examination surveys, 1988–2004. *Clin. Infect. Dis.* **2010**, *50*, 1439–1447. [CrossRef] [PubMed]
16. Cannon, M.J.; Schmid, D.S.; Hyde, T.B. Review of cytomegalovirus seroprevalence and demographic characteristics associated with infection. *Rev. Med. Virol.* **2010**, *20*, 202–213. [CrossRef]
17. Gindes, L.; Teperberg-Oikawa, M.; Sherman, D.; Pardo, J.; Rahav, G. Congenital cytomegalovirus infection following primary maternal infection in the third trimester. *BJOG* **2008**, *115*, 830–835. [CrossRef]
18. Gabrielli, L.; Bonasoni, M.P.; Santini, D.; Piccirilli, G.; Chiereghin, A.; Petrisli, E.; Dolcetti, R.; Guerra, B.; Piccioli, M.; Lanari, M.; et al. Congenital cytomegalovirus infection: Patterns of fetal brain damage. *Clin. Microbiol. Infect.* **2012**, *18*, E419–E427. [CrossRef]
19. Lyutenski, S.; Götz, F.; Giourgas, A.; Majdani, O.; Bültmann, E.; Lanfermann, H.; Lenarz, T.; Giesemann, A.M. Does severity of cerebral MRI lesions in congenital CMV infection correlates with the outcome of cochlear implantation? *Eur. Arch. Otorhinolaryngol.* **2017**, *274*, 1397–1403. [CrossRef]
20. Hawkins-Villarreal, A.; Moreno-Espinosa, A.L.; Eixarch, E.; Marcos, M.A.; Martinez-Portilla, R.J.; Salazar, L.; Garcia-Otero, L.; Lopez, M.; Borrell, A.; Figueras, F.; et al. Blood parameters in fetuses infected with cytomegalovirus according to the severity of brain damage and trimester of pregnancy at cordocentesis. *J. Clin. Virol.* **2019**, *119*, 37–43. [CrossRef]
21. Davis, N.L.; King, C.C.; Kourtis, A.P. Cytomegalovirus infection in pregnancy. *Birth Defects Res.* **2017**, *109*, 336–346. [CrossRef] [PubMed]
22. Kenneson, A.; Cannon, M.J. Review and meta-analysis of the epidemiology of congenital cytomegalovirus (CMV) infection. *Rev. Med. Virol.* **2007**, *17*, 253–276. [CrossRef] [PubMed]
23. Dollard, S.C.; Grosse, S.D.; Ross, D.S. New estimates of the prevalence of neurological and sensory sequelae and mortality associated with congenital cytomegalovirus infection. *Rev. Med. Virol.* **2007**, *17*, 355–363. [CrossRef] [PubMed]
24. Fabbri, E.; Revello, M.G.; Furione, M.; Zavattoni, M.; Lilleri, D.; Tassis, B.; Quarenghi, A.; Rustico, M.; Nicolini, U.; Ferrazzi, E.; et al. Prognostic markers of symptomatic congenital human cytomegalovirus infection in fetal blood. *BJOG* **2011**, *118*, 448–456. [CrossRef] [PubMed]
25. Micallef, S.; Galea, R. CMV encephalitis in an immune-competent patient. *BMJ Case Rep.* **2018**. [CrossRef]
26. Renard, T.; Daumas-Duport, B.; Auffray-Calvier, E.; Bourcier, R.; Desal, H. Cytomegalovirus encephalitis: Undescribed diffusion-weighted imaging characteristics. Original aspects of cases extracted from a retrospective study, and from literature review. *J. Neuroradiol.* **2016**, *43*, 371–377. [CrossRef]
27. Goerig, N.L.; Frey, B.; Korn, K.; Fleckenstein, B.; Überla, K.; Schmidt, M.A.; Dörfler, A.; Engelhorn, T.; Eyüpoglu, I.; Rühle, P.F.; et al. Frequent occurrence of therapeutically reversible CMV-associated encephalopathy during radiotherapy of the brain. *Neuro Oncol.* **2016**, *18*, 1664–1672. [CrossRef]
28. Sierra, A.; de Castro, F.; Del Rio-Hortega, J.; Iglesias-Rozas, J.R.; Garrosa, M.; Kettenmann, H. The "Big-Bang" for Modern Glial Biology: Translation and comments on Pío del Río-Hortega 1919 series of papers on microglia. *Glia* **2016**, *64*, 1801–1840. [CrossRef]
29. Pandey, G.N.; Rizavi, H.S.; Zhang, H.; Bhaumik, R.; Ren, X. Abnormal protein and mRNA expression of inflammatory cytokines in the prefrontal cortex of depressed individuals who died by suicide. *J. Psychiatry Neurosci.* **2018**, *43*, 170192. [CrossRef]

30. Al-Haddad, B.J.S.; Oler, E.; Armistead, B.; Elsayed, N.A.; Weinberger, D.R.; Bernier, R.; Burd, I.; Kapur, R.; Jacobsson, B.; Wang, C.; et al. The fetal origins of mental illness. *Am. J. Obstet. Gynecol.* **2019**, *221*, 549–562. [CrossRef]
31. Zhang, Y.; Träskman-Bendz, L.; Janelidze, S.; Langenberg, P.; Saleh, A.; Constantine, N.; Okusaga, O.; Bay-Richter, C.; Brundin, L.; Postolache, T.T. Toxoplasma gondii immunoglobulin G antibodies and nonfatal suicidal self-directed violence. *J. Clin. Psychiatry.* **2012**, *73*, 1069–1076. [CrossRef] [PubMed]
32. Okusaga, O.; Langenberg, P.; Sleemi, A.; Vaswani, D.; Giegling, I.; Hartmann, A.M.; Konte, B.; Friedl, M.; Groer, M.W.; Yolken, R.H.; et al. Toxoplasma gondii antibody titers and history of suicide attempts in patients with schizophrenia. *Schizophr. Res.* **2011**, *133*, 150–155. [CrossRef] [PubMed]
33. Burgdorf, K.S.; Simonsen, J.; Sundby, A.; Rostgaard, K.; Pedersen, O.B.; Sørensen, E.; Nielsen, K.R.; Bruun, M.T.; Frisch, M.; Edgren, G.; et al. Socio-demographic characteristics of Danish blood donors. *PLoS ONE* **2017**, *12*, e0169112. [CrossRef] [PubMed]
34. Ishii, T.; Hashimoto, E.; Ukai, W.; Kakutani, Y.; Sasaki, R.; Saito, T. Characteristics of attempted suicide by patients with schizophrenia compared with those with mood disorders: A case-controlled study in northern Japan. *PLoS ONE* **2014**, *9*, e96272. [CrossRef] [PubMed]
35. Lopez-Morinigo, J.D.; Fernandes, A.C.; Chang, C.K.; Hayes, R.D.; Broadbent, M.; Stewart, R.; David, A.S.; Dutta, R. Suicide completion in secondary mental healthcare: A comparison study between schizophrenia spectrum disorders and all other diagnoses. *BMC Psychiatry* **2014**, *14*, 213. [CrossRef] [PubMed]
36. Keaton, S.A.; Madaj, Z.B.; Heilman, P.; Smart, L.; Grit, J.; Gibbons, R.; Postolache, T.T.; Roaten, K.; Achtyes, E.D.; Brundin, L. An inflammatory profile linked to increased suicide risk. *J. Affect. Disord.* **2019**, *247*, 57–65. [CrossRef] [PubMed]
37. Black, C.; Miller, B.J. Meta-analysis of cytokines and chemokines in suicidality: Distinguishing suicidal versus nonsuicidal patients. *Biol. Psychiatry* **2015**, *78*, 28–37. [CrossRef]
38. Gananҫa, L.; Oquendo, M.A.; Tyrka, A.R.; Cisneros-Trujillo, S.; Mann, J.J.; Sublette, M.E. The role of cytokines in the pathophysiology of suicidal behavior. *Psychoneuroendocrinology* **2016**, *63*, 296–310. [CrossRef]
39. Wu, W.L.; Hsiao, E.Y.; Yan, Z.; Mazmanian, S.K.; Patterson, P.H. The placental interleukin-6 signaling controls fetal brain development and behavior. *Brain Behav. Immun.* **2017**, *62*, 11–23. [CrossRef]
40. Cheeran, M.C.; Lokensgard, J.R.; Schleiss, M.R. Neuropathogenesis of congenital cytomegalovirus infection: Disease mechanisms and prospects for intervention. *Clin. Microbiol. Rev.* **2009**, *22*, 99–126. [CrossRef]
41. Suzuki, H.; Ohgidani, M.; Kuwano, N.; Chrétien, F.; Lorin de la Grandmaison, G.; Onaya, M.; Tominaga, I.; Setoyama, D.; Kang, D.; Mimura, M.; et al. Suicide and microglia: Recent findings and future perspectives based on human studies. *Front. Cell. Neurosci.* **2019**, *13*, 31. [CrossRef] [PubMed]

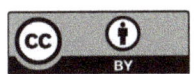

© 2019 by the authors. Licensee MDPI, Basel, Switzerland. This article is an open access article distributed under the terms and conditions of the Creative Commons Attribution (CC BY) license (http://creativecommons.org/licenses/by/4.0/).

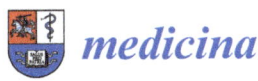

Review

Rational Suicide in Late Life: A Systematic Review of the Literature

Carla Gramaglia [1,2,*], **Raffaella Calati** [3,4] **and Patrizia Zeppegno** [1,2]

1. Institute of Psychiatry, Università degli Studi del Piemonte Orientale, 28100 Novara, Italy; patrizia.zeppegno@med.uniupo.it
2. S.C. Psichiatria, Azienda Ospedaliero Universitaria Maggiore della Carità, 28100 Novara, Italy
3. Department of Psychology, University of Milano-Bicocca, 20126 Milan, Italy; raffaella.calati@gmail.com
4. Nîmes University Hospital, 30029 Nîmes, France
* Correspondence: carla.gramaglia@gmail.com; Tel./Fax: +39-03-2139-0163

Received: 19 August 2019; Accepted: 20 September 2019; Published: 29 September 2019

Abstract: *Background and Objectives*: The complex concept of rational suicide, defined as a well-thought-out decision to die by an individual who is mentally competent, is even more controversial in the case of older adults. *Materials and Methods*: With the aim of better understanding the concept of rational suicide in older adults, we performed a systematic review of the literature, searching PubMed and Scopus databases and eventually including 23 published studies. *Results*: The main related topics emerging from the papers were: depression, self-determination, mental competence; physicians' and population's perspectives; approach to rational suicide; ageism; slippery slope. *Conclusions*: Despite contrasting positions and inconsistencies of the studies, the need to carefully investigate and address the expression of suicidal thoughts in older adults, as well as behaviours suggesting "silent" suicidal attitudes, clearly emerges, even in those situations where there is no diagnosable mental disorder. While premature conclusions about the "rationality" of patients' decision to die should be avoided, the possibility of rational suicide cannot be precluded.

Keywords: rational suicide; old age; late life; aging; ageism

1. Introduction

Suicide is a global phenomenon accounting for 800,000 deaths worldwide every year [1]. Considering the global aging trends in the world and that suicide rates increase with age, suicide in older adults cannot be neglected [2–4]. Older adults account for a disproportionately high number of suicide deaths because they are more successful at committing suicide compare to younger adults [5].

In older age there is a high risk of unrecognized and untreated psychiatric illnesses [6,7]. In particular, depression is the most common disorder and the most important risk factor associated with late life suicide [3,8–10]. However, most depressed older adults do not become suicidal. Furthermore, approximately 55% of late life suicides are associated with physical illness [3,4], and older people and those with chronic/terminal illness may not have psychiatric comorbidity. Physical illness is more likely to eventually lead to suicidal behaviour when it causes functional disabilities threatening the individual's independence, autonomy and dignity, quality of and pleasure with life, sense of meaning, usefulness and purpose in life, perceived personal value and self-esteem [11–13].

Aging may lead individuals to think back about their lives and to experience either feelings of integrity (if they feel their life has been meaningful) or despair (if they are unable to find meaning and achievement in their life) [14]. Moreover, notwithstanding what they have achieved in their life, older adults have to face changes, which are usually losses, in the context of several domains including health, employment, and relationships. Thus, the aging individual is compelled to go through grieving experiences and redefinitions of one's identity [13] which, if unsuccessful, lead to a damage of the individual's sense of self. The old age individual's skills in redefining their physical selves and integrating changes depends on their "historical" attribution of meaning to their body [13,15]. Amery defined aging as an incurable disease, where "the body becomes more and more mass and less and less energy. This mass ... is the new, enemy self", and "alien and authentically adverse self" which is opposed to the "self of the past"[16]: this sense of internal division between one's sick and healthy selves, with the first being perceived as "alien" by the latter, may lead the healthy self to wish the destruction of the sick one [13,15].

Furthermore, the current historical period is one marked by many new opportunities (including good hygienic conditions, availability of clean water, fresh food, quality public health, progress in medical knowledge and available treatments, starting from antibiotics) which have allowed a rapid increase of life expectancy and longevity, but also by the difficulties and ambiguities in facing what these opportunities have brought about. Life support technologies currently enable the prolongment of critically ill patients' life, often beyond a point where it can be experienced as meaningful and desirable [17]. Therefore, since living longer does not necessarily mean living a high-quality life, the need to balance benefits and harms of curative and, even more, palliative therapies, especially for painful, terminal illnesses, has opened new topics of legal, moral, and ethical concern.

In recent years, there has been much discussion (not only in the scientific community) about suicide and what has been named "rational suicide" in older adults. It is described as "rational" an action which is "sensible, appropriate, in keeping with one's fundamental interests, and perhaps even admirable"[18]. Rationality means being capable of deliberating, with no coercion, according to one's own values and purposes in life [19], and that motives and plans for a certain decision have been thoroughly explored, as well as alternative choices [20]. Therefore, rational suicide may be defined as a sane, well-thought-out and fairly stable decision by an individual who is mentally competent, and who is capable of reasoning and choosing the best alternative among the many available with no ambivalence (see Table 1 for the main definitions and criteria to define the construct of rational suicide).

Table 1. Definitions and criteria for rational suicide.

	Definition/Criteria of Rational Suicide
Siegel [21]	Realistic assessment of the situation on behalf of a person whose mental processes are not impaired by either psychological illness or severe emotional distress. The motivational basis for the decision could be understandable on behalf of uninvolved observers.
Cheung et al. [2]	Add further details about Siegel criterion (3): (1) The person understood the terminal nature of her/his condition. (2) The person consciously disengaged from treatment. (3) The person communicated the desire or made preparations to end her/his life. (4) A triggering event heightened a hopeless situation.
Werth & Cobia [22]	Presence of an unremitting hopeless condition (such as terminal illness, severe pain, both physical and psychological, deteriorating conditions, no longer acceptable quality of life, etc). The decision is a free choice. The decision results from a sound decision making process including the consultation with a mental health professional, and with objective and significant others; a non-impulsive assessment of alternatives, of the possible impact of the decision on significant others, and of the congruence of the decision with the individual's personal values.
Valente & Trainor [19]	Rational decisions reflect careful planning and consideration of adequate information (e.g., complete and accurate medical facts); preparations (e.g., wills, funeral arrangements); consideration of effect on others, treatment options and alternatives.
Motto [23]	A rational decision should be realistic (i.e., should be made after a realistic assessment of the individual's situation and after gaining full knowledge of options and consequences) and have minimal ambivalence (i.e., a decision should not be made on the basis of a transient desire and should not be inconsistent with the individual's longstanding and fundamental values).
Diekstra [24]	Enduring wish to die in a person with a condition of enduring unbearable physical and/or emotional pain, no hope for improvement. The person, who is not mentally disturbed, makes a free will decision which would not cause "unnecessary or preventable harm" to others.
Humphry [25]	"Considered decision" on behalf of a mature adult individual, after reasonable medical help has been sought and the treating physician has been informed. A will should be made and a note should be left. The suicide should not involve others criminally.
Weber [26]	Two meanings of right to die: - right to refuse life-sustaining treatment; - an "affirmative right to obtain death-a right to suicide".
Graber [27]	A reasonable appraisal of the situation reveals that one would be really better off dead.

The concept of rational suicide is controversial and difficult to define, so that some suicidologists and psychologists consider it as an oxymoron. The debate about this topic is even more complicated by emerging and complex to define concepts such as those of "good" or "gentle death", and of "silent suicide", defined as the intention to kill oneself by nonviolent means such as refusal of food and liquids or noncompliance with essential medical treatment. Such means of promoting one's death causes ambiguity in medical, clinical, personal, cultural, ethical, religious and historical interpretations [28]. Moreover, the concept of rational suicide is obviously linked to the debate about the hot topic of euthanasia, physician assisted death (PAD) and physician assisted suicide (PAS) (i.e., if suicide can be rational, then the right-to-die should be legal and regulated).

Given the ongoing debate about the possibility that a "rational suicide" exists, the concern represented by older adults' suicide and the world population aging trend, we performed a systematic review of the literature about rational suicide in late life, with the primary aim to offer an overview and better understanding of the concept of rational suicide in older adults through a description of the main related topics emerged from the literature.

2. Materials and Methods

We searched PubMed and Scopus databases from inception to April 16th and 19th 2019, respectively, with the following search keywords: rational AND suicid* AND (elderly OR older*). Two of the Authors (C.G., R.C.) reviewed and screened eligible articles according to the PRISMA (Preferred Reporting Items for Systematic Reviews and Meta-Analyses) flow diagram [29]. Any disagreement among reviewers was solved through discussion and with the supervision of the third Author (P.Z.). Studies were included if: (1) they focused on rational suicide defined according to one or more of the criteria mentioned in Table 1; (2) they focused on or included/mentioned older adults. To ensure the most complete reporting of the available literature about the topic, we decided to include all available study designs.

Studies were excluded if: (1) they were written in languages other than English; (2) their full-text was not available; (3) they were book chapters, commentaries and editorials/letters to the editor; (4) they were focused on euthanasia, PAD and PAS.

For each study, we extracted: year, design, sample features, used rating scales, reasons mentioned for rational suicide, rational suicide criteria and/or definition, main results, and conclusions.

3. Results

3.1. Main (Quantitative) Features of the Included Studies

The search retrieved 144 references; 24 full text articles were assessed for eligibility (see Figure 1 for the flow diagram); 1 full text article was not available for the assessment. We eventually included 23 published studies in the review.

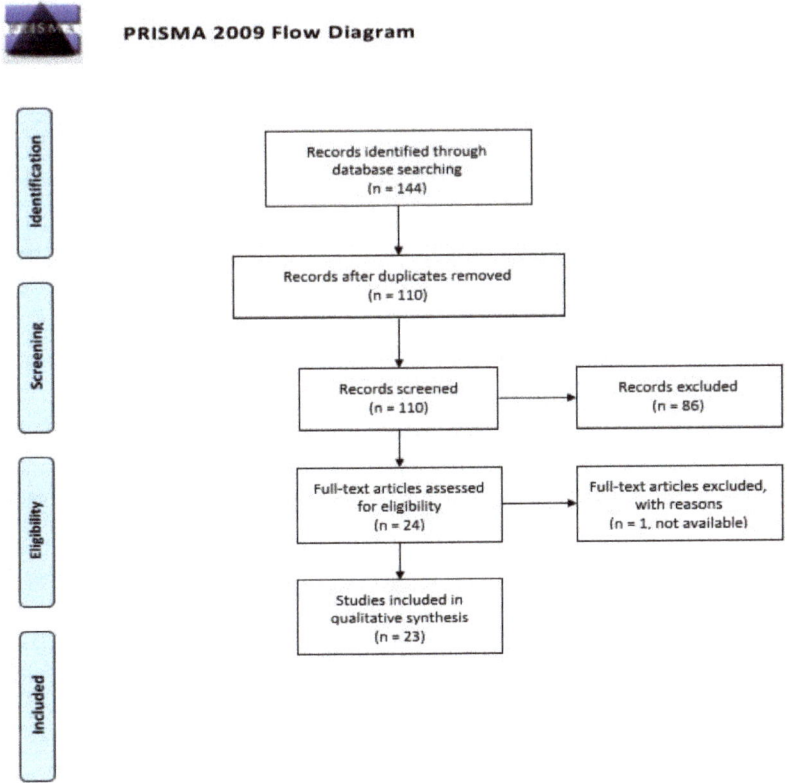

Figure 1. PRISMA 2009 Flow Diagram [29].

The data extracted for each of the studies are described in Table 2, where articles are presented in alphabetical order.

Table 2. Summary of the included articles in alphabetical order.

Author, Year	Perspective/Approach	Sample Features/Specialists	Rating Scales	Empirical Studies Including Data		RS Criteria and/or Definition	Main Results and Conclusions
				Topics Covered/Reasons Mentioned for RS			
Cheung et al. 2017 [2]	Focus on the comparison between older people with and without terminal cancer who died by suicide, and analysis of motives for suicide. Hypothesis: in older people with terminal cancer, suicide can be considered a rational choice rather than the result of depression.	Source: Coroner records about suicides in ≥ 65-year-old 07/2007–12/2012, with available data about terminal cancer, N = 214, 74.3% males, 60.7% aged 65–79-year-old N = 23 (10.7%) terminal cancer.	n.a.	- Burden - Control (loss of) - Dependence - Dignity - Functional disability - Pain - Physical illness - Pleasure with life (loss of) - QoL - Sense of usefulness, purpose, value (loss of)		Siegel, 1986 [17] (3rd characteristic: a motivational basis that would be understandable to uninvolved observers) Werth & Cobia, 1995 [22]	- Older patients with terminal cancer who died by suicide were less likely depressed and to have had previous contact with mental health services. - 82.6% of terminal cancer cases had a motivational basis for suicide, understandable to uninvolved observers, due to physical (pain, functional disability) or psychological suffering. - Underdiagnosis of depression in patients with terminal cancer? - Choice to end one's life as a rational act to alleviate suffering?
Fortin et al. 2001 [30]	Focus on suicide prevention. Health care personnel (not mental health professionals) performing assessment.	N = 66 French-Caucasian older adults (age range between 69 and 96 y.o.) with no cognitive deficit, from 7 long-term facilities. N = 11 suicidal (N = 7 males). N = 55 non suicidal (N = 22 matched for age, gender, civil status).	PAQ GDS	- Control (loss of) - Decreased self-esteem - Helplessness - Hopelessness - Losses (physical, psychological, emotional, social, environmental) - Pain - QoL - Relationship problems - Satisfaction		Werth & Cobia (1995) [22], mentioned (but not used)	- No difference in self-determination between older adults with/without SI. - Differences on social subscale: SI have less consideration of own behaviour's impact on others and less satisfaction with relations with children and family relationships. - SI more depressed than non-SI. - Debate on RS warrants research on self-determination.

Table 2. Cont.

Author, Year	Perspective/Approach	Sample Features/Specialists	Rating Scales	Topics Covered/Reasons Mentioned for RS	RS Criteria and/or Definition	Main Results and Conclusions
Gibbs et al. 2009 [31]	Focus on problem solving strategies, closely related to the topic of suicidality in old age.	N = 64 > 60-year-old MMSE >18 - N = 18 Depressed elderly with past SA. - N = 27 Depressed elderly never suicidal. - N = 19 Non-depressed elderly.	SPSI-R MMSE HAM-D BHS B-SIS SIS B-SLS CIRS-G	- Dependence - Loss - Physical illness	n.s.	- Depressed elderly SA perceived problem solving as dysfunctional and deficient compared to depressed non-attempters and non-depressed elderly: problems perceived more negatively and approached more impulsively and carelessly. This is in contrast with the common clinical view of late-life SA and those who die by suicide as being non-impulsive. - Both depressed groups compared to non-depressed elderly had lower rational and positive problem solving. - Depressed SA showed higher avoidant style than non-depressed elderly. - Lifetime diagnosis of SUD predicted lower total problem-solving score, higher negative problem orientation/impulsivity, and avoidance scores.
Uncapher and Arean 2000 [32]	To determine the influence of patients' age on primary care physician recognition of suicidal symptoms and the willingness to treat the suicidal patient.	N = 342 physicians (63% response rate), of whom N = 215 primary care physicians, asked to assess 2 vignettes of depressed suicidal patient, either geriatric, retired, age 78 y.o. (N = 100), or young, employed, 38 y.o. (N = 115).	21-item Suicidal Patient Treatment Scale	n.s.	n.s.	- Physicians recognized depression (99%) and suicidal risk (94%). - Physicians were less willing to treat the older patient, feeling that his SI was rational and normal. - Possible age bias?

Table 2. *Cont.*

Author, Year	Perspective/Approach	Sample Features/Specialists	Rating Scales	Topics Covered/Reasons Mentioned for RS	RS Criteria and/or Definition	Main Results and Conclusions
Van Wijngaarden et al. 2016 [33]	Qualitative in-depth interview study aimed at a phenomenological characterization of the phenomenon "life is completed and no longer worth living".	N = 25, > 82 y.o. N = 11 males form the Netherlands, ideating on self-chosen death. Inclusion criteria: (1) considered their lives to be 'completed'; (2) suffered from the prospect of living on; (3) current wish to die; (4) 70 y.o. or older; (5) not terminally ill; (6) considered themselves to be mentally competent; (7) considered their death wish reasonable. N = 23 members of RTD organizations.	Interview HADS	- Burden - Control (loss of) - Dependence - Dignity (loss of) - Interpersonal theory of suicide: thwarted belongingness, perceived burdensomness - Loneliness - Meaning - Pain - QoL	n.s.	- Themes: detachment & attachment; rational & non-rational considerations; taking control & lingering uncertainty; resisting interference & longing for support; legitimacy & illegitimacy. - Rationality versus inner uncontrolled compulsion. - Ambiguities and ambivalence present after a putatively rational decision: need to develop careful policy and support for older people. - Results question the concept of rational suicide as an autonomous, free decision without pressure.
Winterrowd et al. 2017 [34]	To examine beliefs/opinions (most likely precipitants and protectors) and attitudes about older adults' suicide, in a cultural perspective.	N = 255 older adults (86% European American), 70.95 y.o. mean age, 38% males. N = 281 younger adults (81% European American), 19.04 y.o. mean age, 30% males.	Ad hoc attitudes Scale Personal Attribute Questionnaire-Short Form	n.s.	n.s.	- Precipitants: health problems, mostly in older adults; rational/courageous suicide, admissible (56.7%). - Most favourable attitude about older adult suicide: older adults, persons with more education, persons not identifying with a religion, persons with a history of suicidality. - Older adults suicide viewed as more admissible by males and with more sympathy by females. - Protectors: religiosity in older adults (21.1%); supportive relationships (37.9%) in younger adults. - Mental health care believed to play a preventative role by 6.7% respondents.

Table 2. Cont.

Author, Year	Perspective/Approach	Sample Features/Specialists	Rating Scales	Case Studies Specifically Focused on Late Life Rational Suicide		Main Results and Conclusions
				Topics Covered/Reasons Mentioned for RS	RS Criteria and/or Definition	
Balasubramaniam 2018 [13]	Case presentation: 72 y.o. male, retired, widowed, with adenocarcinoma.	Geriatricians Psychogeriatricians	MCAS (used) DDRS and SATHD (mentioned)	Ageism Control (loss of) Dependence Frailty Gerontophobia Loss QoL Sense of identity/Sense of self (loss of)	-	- Geriatricians increasingly encounter older adults expressing the desire to end their lives, who may have medical illnesses (not necessarily terminal ones), but no diagnosable mental illness. - Is the absence of a diagnostic category to describe a mental state in which suicide appears like the best option a flaw in nosology? - Is RS a rational entity that will be increasingly encountered as views about health, choice, and control continue to evolve?
Lerner 1995 [35]	Case Story of a Couple and Review of Humphry's Book Final Exit	n.s.	n.a.	Autonomy (loss of) Terminal illness Terminal old age	n.s.	- Ageism and slippery slope. - Ambiguities surrounding elder suicide. - Need to approach elder suicide in the context of individual life experiences.
Simon 1989 [7]	Clinical/legal issues of silent S + 2 cases (clinical) + case law examples.	Clinicians	n.a.	Autonomy (loss of) Factors including psychological, social, ethical, cultural, economic and situational Losses Medical complaints	n.s.	- Silent S: by non-violent means as self-starvation or non-compliance with essential medical treatments. - Frequently unrecognized because of underdiagnosed depression and/or interjection of personal belief systems of healthcare providers and/or family members. - Cognitive and affective aspects of decision making. - Mental competency impaired (de jure or de facto) by depression: "Premature conclusions that the patient has made a 'rational' decision to die must be avoided"; anyway, "certainly every elderly patient who is depressed is not incompetent". - Treatment: ECT, antidepressants, psychotherapy.

Table 2. Cont.

Author, Year	Perspective/Approach	Sample Features/Specialists	Rating Scales	Case Studies Specifically Focused on Late Life Rational Suicide		Main Results and Conclusions
				Topics Covered/Reasons Mentioned for RS	RS Criteria and/or Definition	
Wand et al. 2016 [36]	2 cases discussed in the light of the importance of a narrative and bio-psycho-social approach to the management of the wish to die.	Psychiatrists Psychogeriatricians	MCAT	Autonomy (loss of) Burden Control (loss of) Coping strategies Dependence Disability External support Helplessness Hopelessness Loss of purpose/meaning/role in life QoL Scared of institutional care Tiredness of living	Battin 1984 [37] Conwell & Caine, 1991 [38]	- Open question about the possible differences between people expressing a wish to die and SA. Does a continuum exist, from wish to die, to SA, to S? - Rationality is probably dimensional rather than dichotomous (Conwell & Caine, 1991). - Requests for euthanasia may occur in older people in the absence of a significant mood disorder. - Ageism and medical paternalism. - Relevant topics: Narrative formulation; Crafting an advance care directive; Exploration of spiritual issues; empathic ongoing care/support; Support both for patients and families; Social interventions.

Author, Year	Perspective/Approach	Sample Features/Specialists	Rating Scales	Case Studies Not Specifically Focused on Late Life Rational Suicide (But Mentioning It in the Text)		Main Results and Conclusions
				Topics Covered/Reasons Mentioned for RS	RS Criteria and/or Definition	
Fontana 2002 [39]	Historical and philosophical perspective + case description. RTD, PAS, euthanasia mentioned; Hemlock society mentioned.	Nurses	n.a.	Autonomy (loss of) Control (loss of) Dignity Loss of meaning/purpose in life Pain QoL Self-determination	Siegel, 1986 [17] Werth, 1995 [22]	- Good death as a right. - Problem of having no position and no guiding principle from AMA and ANA. - Implications for the meaning of care (in nursing).
Karlinsky et al. 1988 [40]	Psychological, ethical, legal issues + 2 cases, one advanced age, one terminal illness; euthanasia mentioned; Hemlock Society mentioned.	n.s.	n.a.	Competency Control (loss of) Dependence Disability, physical Mental state/psychiatric illness QoL	n.s.	- Contradictions between the principles of patients' autonomy and physicians' responsibility. - Living will.

Table 2. Cont.

Author, Year	Perspective/Approach	Sample Features/Specialists	Rating Scales	Case Studies Not Specifically Focused on Late Life Rational Suicide (But Mentioning It in the Text)		Main Results and Conclusions
				Topics Covered/Reasons Mentioned for RS	RS Criteria and/or Definition	
Rich 2004 [28]	Historical, ethical + case description of chronic AIDS; PAS, euthanasia mentioned; Hemlock Society mentioned; VSED and terminal sedation mentioned.	Nurses	n.a.	Escape from life Terminal illness Disability, permanent Autonomy (loss of) Pain	Siegel, 1986 [17] Werth, 1999 [41] Werth & Cobia, 1995 [22]	- Ethics of care: "principles alone do not provide a comprehensive basis for the most important ethical decisions". - Slippery slope. - Autonomy versus beneficence principles. - Meaning of a caring relationship (exploration of feelings – including caregivers'; meaningful communication; thoughtful decision making). - Lack of guidelines from AMA and ANA.

Author, Year	Perspective/Approach	Sample Features/Specialists	Rating Scales	Opinion Studies Specifically Focused on Late Life Rational Suicide		Main Results and Conclusions
				Topics Covered/Reasons Mentioned for RS	RS Criteria and/or Definition	
Conwell & Caine 1991 [38]	Critical position	Psychiatrists Psychogeriatricians Researchers Consultants	n.a.	Ageism Burden Physical illness QoL	n.s.	- Poor attention paid to the effects of psychiatric illness on rational decision making in the context of the debate on RS. - Personal biases possibly affecting the determination of a suicidal person's "rationality": about aging, old age, psychological effects of chronic disease. - Suicide in the absence of treatable affective illness is uncommon; critical depressive illness precludes rational decision making. - Differential diagnosis: depressed mood versus sadness developing as a natural response to serious illness. - Peculiar presentation of major depressive illness in old age, reduced use of mental health services on behalf of elderly.

Table 2. Cont.

Author, Year	Perspective/Approach	Sample Features/ Specialists	Rating Scales	Topics Covered/Reasons Mentioned for RS	RS Criteria and/or Definition	Main Results and Conclusions
Gallagher-Thompson &Osgood 1997 [42]	Overview of epidemiology of late life S, demographics and risk factors, assessment, RS.	Healthcare professionals	BHS MSSI BDI GDS SCID	Autonomy (loss of) Control (loss of) Dignity (loss of) Disability Hopelessness Loss of meaning in life Losses Pain Poor self-esteem QoL Terminal illness	Diekstra, 1986 [24] Motto, 1972 [23] Battin, 1991 [43] Humphry, 1992 [25] Werth & Cobia, 1995 [22]	- Risk factors for old age S: > 60 y.o., Caucasian, divorced/widowed, no longer employed, poor health, depressed or not, alcohol, access to gun, reduced self-esteem, history of mental illness, history of S, poor relationships. - Arguments in favour: philosophy, autonomy, meaning in life. - Proposed interventions to reduce SI and increase QoL: medication, ECT, support groups.
Humphry 1992 [25]	Position of the leader of the National Hemlock Society, mentioning euthanasia and PAS + case narrative.	n.s.	n.a.	Choice (loss of) Control (loss of) "Living death"Pain/suffering, both physical and emotional Terminal illness	n.s.	- "Suicide and assisted suicide carried out in the face of terminal illness causing unbearable suffering should be ethically and legally acceptable". - Slippery slope.
Moore 1993 [44]	Historical perspective and discussion of supportive and opposing arguments; implications for nursing. "Old age in our society needs to be viewed once again as a valued status, rather than a cursed disease or a burden".	Nurses Psychologists	n.a.	Burden Control (loss of) Lack of satisfying role Meaning (loss of)	Weber, 1988b [26] Graber, 1981 [27]	- Supportive: right to self-determination; evil of needless suffering; Battin's 17 considerations for assessment. - Opposing: ageism; slippery slope. Having no alternative but suicide raises doubts about the rationality of older adults' decision. - Individual life histories, not aging, are critical for the understanding of suicide in later years.
Prado 2015 [45]	Philosophical and bioethical perspective; discussion of the author's position.	n.s.	n.a.	Conditions diminishing the individual as a person, irremediable Dependence Hopeless medical situations Irreversible deterioration Pain	n.s.	- "Life is not itself an unconditional good", and sheer organic survival is not an absolute value. - "Whatever the condition of our bodies, once our minds deteriorate beyond a certain point, we cease to exist as the person we are". - Proposed objections to S/SA: moral, religious, cultural, social, legal.

Table 2. *Cont.*

Author, Year	Perspective/Approach	Sample Features/Specialists	Rating Scales	Opinion Studies Specifically Focused on Late Life Rational Suicide		Main Results and Conclusions
				Topics Covered/Reasons Mentioned for RS	RS Criteria and/or Definition	
Richards 2016 [46]	Empirical/theoretical overview to synthesize knowledge, including existential questions about the perception of complete life or tiredness of life.	n.s.	n.a.	Burden Control (loss of) Dependence Disability, functional Illness, chronic Loneliness Loss of meaning/purpose in life Losses Pain, suffering Personality and coping strategies Psychological issues (depression, cognitive decline) QoL Social isolation Tiredness of life	Werth, 1999 [41] Battin, 1991 [43] McCue & Balasubramaniam, 2017 [47]	- Not all SI or planning for S should be unquestioningly pathologized. - Decision making is not a purely cognitive process. - Not all motivating factors for old age RS are open to be remedied. - Importance of end of life care context in which older people find themselves.
Ruckenbauer et al. 2007 [48]	Critical revision of RS. Tension between medical care for patients and patients' autonomy.	Physicians	n.a.	Burden Conflict Illness Loss Pain Traditional family structures falling apart	n.s.	- Suicide as symptom of individually and/or socially conditioned lack of freedom, rather than of sovereign self-determination. - Underestimation of depression and suicidal potential in old age. - Cult of youthfulness versus old age, associated with weakness, deficiency, increased health costs.

Table 2. *Cont.*

Author, Year	Perspective/Approach	Sample Features/Specialists	Rating Scales	Topics Covered/Reasons Mentioned for RS	RS Criteria and/or Definition	Main Results and Conclusions
				Opinion studies not Specifically Focused on Late Life Rational Suicide (but Mentioning it in the Text)		
Battin 1991 [43]	S not interpreted as evidence of depression or mental illness; meaning and motivation.	Mental health professionals	n.a.	Terminal illness Disability, severe and permanent Advanced old age	Motto, 1972 (mentioned) [23]	- Presentation and discussion of 17 reasons which should be explored to understand whether S would be rational or not. - "[….] respectful and humane way" to approach "persons who, in a society now beginning to consider S as a rational and even responsible way of avoiding the degradations of terminal illness, severe permanent disability, or extreme old age, wish to explore this option with a trained and insightful professional".
Clark 1992 [49]	Overview of S and terminal illness, PAS, RTD and euthanasia mentioned; Hemlock Society mentioned. Critical position versus the "understandable reasons" for contemplating S.	Mental health professionals General internists Family physicians	n.a.	Dependence Deteriorating health Disability Helplessness Hopelessness Isolation Loneliness Outliving family members Pain Poverty Severe illness	n.s.	- The so called "understandable reasons" for S rarely stand alone, with no coexisting psychiatric illness, as causes of suicidal thinking. - Almost all persons who die by S evidence symptoms of major psychiatric illness. - Features of depressive illness often overlooked. - Possibility of RS not precluded, but there is likely a strong cultural bias to overlook the "forces and motives implicated in cases of S by older persons". - The question of mental competence to opt for S.

Table 2. *Cont.*

| Author, Year | Perspective/Approach | Sample Features/Specialists | Rating Scales | Opinion studies not Specifically Focused on Late Life Rational Suicide (but Mentioning it in the Text) |||
				Topics Covered/Reasons Mentioned for RS	RS Criteria and/or Definition	Main Results and Conclusions
Siegel 1982 [21]	Evolving societal values concerning death and S, RTD, RTS; Hemlock Society mentioned.	Clinicians	n.a.	QoL Pain Loss of meaning in life Lack of support Self-determination Control (loss of)	Hoche's "Balance sheet suicide"	- Living will. - Conflictual and ambivalent nature of SA. - Intervention appropriate if (1) the individual is not completely resolved in the decision to die (conflict, ambivalence); (2) the individual does not seem to be realistically appraising his/her problems or prospects for the future.

Legend: AMA: American Medical Association; ANA: American Nursing Association; BDI: Beck Depression Inventory; BHS: Beck Hopelessness Scale; B-SIS: Beck Scale for Suicidal Ideation; B-SLS: Beck Suicide Lethality Scale; CIRS-G: Cumulative Illness Rating Scale adapted for Geriatrics; DDRS: Desire for Death Rating Scale; GDS: Geriatric Depression Scale; HADS: Hospital Anxiety and Depression Scale; HAM-D: Hamilton Depression Rating Scale; MCAS: Montreal Cognitive Assessment Scale; MCAT: Montreal Cognitive Assessment Test; MMSE: Mini-Mental State Examination; MSSI: Modified Scale for Suicidal Ideation; n.a.: not applicable; n.s.: not specified; PAQ: Psychological Autonomy Questionnaire; PAS: Physician Assisted Suicide; QoL: Quality of Life; RS: Rational Suicide; RTD: Right to Die; RTS: Right to Suicide; S: suicide; SA: suicide attempt/suicide attempters; SATHD: Schedule of Attitudes Towards Hastened Death; SCID: Structured Clinical Interview for DSM; SI: suicidal ideation/individuals with suicidal ideation; SIS: Suicide Intent Scale; SPSI-R: Social Problem Solving Inventory – Short Version; SUD: Substance Use Disorder; VSED: voluntary stopping of eating and drinking; y.o.: years old.

Among the included articles, 6 were original papers [2,30–34], with different designs and aims: 1 was based on coroner records of suicides in older people with and without terminal cancer, and investigated motives for rational suicide [2]; 2 assessed suicidal and non-suicidal older adults, one with a specific focus on self-determination [30] and one on problem solving strategies [31]; 1 surveyed primary care physicians and the impact of patients' age on their ability in recognizing suicidal symptoms and willingness to treat patients [32]; 1 used qualitative in-depth interviews to assess older adults ideating on self-chosen death [33]; 1 examined older and younger adults' beliefs and attitudes about late life suicide [37].

Of these six articles, 2 referred to specific criteria or definitions for rational suicide [2,30], and only one out of these two actually used them [2]; in both cases Werth & Cobia's criteria were mentioned, and Cheung also mentioned Siegel's criteria; 1 did not mention rating scales [2].

Four out of the six studies explored and mentioned several reasons for rational suicide [2,30,31,33], with the concept of loss being explicitly or implicitly referred to in all these 4 studies. The following topics were mentioned: control, dependence, disability/illness, pain, quality of life (QoL) (3 studies); burden, dignity, loss of pleasure/meaning in life (2 studies) (see Table 2 for more details).

Eleven of the studies described in Table 2 did not include research data, but were specifically focused on old age rational suicide [7,13,25,35,36,38,42,44–46,48]: 5 included case(s) descriptions [7,13,25,35,36]; 7 specified the professionals involved in end of life and rational suicide issues.

Criteria for rational suicide and rating scales were mentioned respectively by 3 [13,36,42] and 4 [36,42,44,46] of these studies. Battin's and Werth/Werth & Cobia were the most frequently reported criteria for rational suicide. Regarding motives for rational suicide, the most frequently mentioned ones were: loss, including loss of meaning and purpose (9 studies); burden (5 studies); control (5 studies); pain (5 studies); QoL (5 studies); autonomy (4 studies); dependence (4 studies) (see Table 2 for more details).

The concepts of ageism and slippery slope effect were discussed by 2 [13,38] and 3 [25,35,44] studies, respectively.

Last, 6 papers were not specifically focused on late life rational suicide but mentioned it [21,28,39,40,43,49]; 3 included case(s) descriptions; all but one[40] specified the professionals involved in end of life issues. Four of these six studies [21,28,39,43] mentioned criteria for the definition of rational suicide: Motto's [23]; Siegel's [21] and Werth's [41]; Werth & Cobia's [22]; Hoche's "Balance sheet suicide"[21]. Among the reasons for rational suicide, loss (including loss of meaning) was implicitly or explicitly mentioned by all papers; other reasons included: pain (4 studies), disability (4 studies), control (3 studies), QoL (3 studies), dependence (2 studies), autonomy (1 study) (see Table 2 for more details).

All but one of these six papers [43] mentioned the Hemlock Society and either euthanasia, PAD, PAS, right to die; 2 [21,40] mentioned the Living Will.

3.2. Main Topics Covered in the Included Studies

The main topics emerged from the papers included in the review were: depression, self-determination, mental competence; physicians' and population's perspectives; approach to rational suicide; ageism; slippery slope.

Furthermore, Table 3 briefly summarizes arguments in favour versus arguments opposing rational suicide emerging from the included studies.

Table 3. Arguments in favour and opposing rational suicide.

Arguments in Favour of Rational Suicide	Arguments Opposing Rational Suicide
Moral right to self-determination [33]	Should death wishes, and ideation and action aimed at deliberately ending one's life ever be considered as "rational"?
Needless suffering [33]	Ageism: old age individuals as a burden; death as a solution for insoluble age-related suffering [12].
Exerting control over one's death: satisfaction and empowerment.	Slippery slope: from right to die to social obligation to die [9].
Suicidal ideation and behaviour may be the logical and understandable outcome of a balance sheet where death becomes preferable to life [33].	Is suicide *per se* an evidence of mental instability? [33] Having suicidal ideation is often the very reason why an individual is classified as having a mental illness.
Suicide can be a serious and legitimate answer to the individual's existential situation, which should not be dismissed as a depressive symptom [20]. A history of mood disorder (as well as of any other mental illness) does not mean that the individual's decision-making capacity is impaired and should be questioned forever [50,51].	Suicide itself is an emotional condition precluding the possibility of rationality: the suicidal individual is usually not capable to consider other option than suicide to a condition of perceived intolerable misery. One would rather live, if a better solution than suicide was at hand [22,52–55].

3.3. Depression, Self-Determination, and Mental Competence

Though in different ways and from different perspectives, almost all the included articles underscored ambiguities and possible biases regarding old age rational suicide. The point which is most discussed is the possible underestimation of depression in old age patients, either terminally ill or not, and its impact on patients' self-determination and mental competence. Actually, the current nosology includes suicidal ideation and attempts as symptoms of either major depressive episodes and of borderline personality disorder. Thus, the main emerging and unresolved question is whether suicidal ideation and attempt in late life should be always treated as symptoms of a psychiatric disorder or not.

The results about depression in suicidal older adults in the studies we assessed are mixed; while [2] found that among older patients who died by suicide, those with terminal cancer were less likely than those without to be depressed and to have had previous contact with mental health services [30] reported a greater likelihood of depression in elderly with suicidal ideation than in those with no such ideation. These two studies pointed to the question whether or not underdiagnosis of depression is an issue in older patients' suicide, and to the importance of assessing self-determination in the context of the rational suicide debate, respectively.

Consistent with the debate about decisions relying both on judgments and affective states [50], poorer problem-solving skills were found in depressed elderly suicide attempters, compared to depressed non-attempters and non-depressed elderly, in contrast with the commonplace belief that suicide attempt in late life would be non-impulsive [31]. Moreover, considering ambivalence, ambiguities and the contrast between rationality and inner uncontrolled compulsion in elderly ideating on self-chosen death, Van Wijngaarden et al. [33] indings seemed to question the concept of rational suicide as an autonomous, free decision without pressure.

Briefly, what emerges from the studies we assessed is that underdiagnosis of depression in old age and especially in terminal illness is a relevant problem [56–58] ecause it can be difficult to differentiate depressive disorders from old age-related cognitive impairment and from the normal emotional responses of a person coping with a terminal illness [59,60]. On the other hand, not all suicidal individuals are depressed and mental illness per se does not imply that the individual's self-determination and competency are compromised. So, even though a careful assessment of every single situation is mandatory, not every suicidal ideation and/or planning should be "unquestioningly" pathologized. Last, an approach focused on the concept of "understandability" of suicidal ideation and/or behaviour has been suggested as potentially more meaningful and useful than that of rationality, because an approach based on rationality might lead to overlooking the expressive and emotional meaning of the wish to die [52].

3.4. Views of Rational Suicide: Physicians' and Population's Perspectives

Two of the original studies assessed focused on views about rational suicide, on behalf of physicians [32] and of older and younger adults [34].

The first study found that primary care physicians' skills in recognizing depression and suicidal risk in late life were excellent, nonetheless physicians were less willing to treat older patients, likely due to an age bias leading them to consider suicide intent as rational and normal in that age group [32].

In the general population, a more favorable attitude towards late life suicide was found on behalf of older adults compared to younger adults. When asked about possible protective factors for late life suicide, interestingly, only a small percentage of respondents believed that mental health care could play a preventive role [34]. It is not clear whether this last result reflects mistrust in the possibility of suicidal individual to receive help, or rather the general population's actual belief that late life suicide is not a clinical issue. Mankind's history has witnessed changing views about death and suicide, which in clinical contexts have both turned out to be something which should be always prevented, fought and avoided; this is linked to the topic of the principles of autonomy versus beneficence, and of patients' autonomy and physicians' responsibility [28,40]. Conflicts inevitably surround the approach to rational suicide also from this standpoint, starting from the ethical principle guiding healthcare professionals, who should respect patients' autonomy as well as safeguarding their lives. On the other hand, the need of a reflection on the meaning and ethics of care in late life and end of life in the current society has been suggested [28,39].

3.5. Approach to Rational Suicide

A careful assessment of patients, a thorough and accurate investigation of the meaning of their attitudes towards end of life, and the development of appropriate supportive strategies to face the new emerging needs in the care of old age patients are described by most of the included papers.

It is clearly underscored that each situation and the actual meaning of the wish to die should be evaluated in the context of individual life experience and histories, which are critical elements for the understanding of rational suicide [2,35,44].

The position described by most of the articles reviewed is an "interlocutory" one, encouraging a thorough exploration of reasons for suicide in the context of a "respectful and humane" relationship between patient and "a trained and insightful professional" [43], based on the belief that most elderly persons "readily discuss their suicidal feelings and intentions and are glad to be able to share their thoughts with someone who cares enough to ask"[61]. Exploration of reasons and meaning of suicidal ideation and/or attempt is particularly important when it clearly emerges a conflictual and ambivalent nature of the decision to die, and when the individual is not realistically appraising her/his problems and prospects [21].

The approach to rational suicide should go beyond the mere assessment of the presence of a mood disorder, and address the whole range of issues possibly contributing to the individual's wish to die, in order to offer possible targets for interventions, and allow the implementation of approaches aimed at increasing QoL or decreasing pain, distress and suffering, which may eventually lead to a reduction of suicidal ideation [30,42,46,62,63].

3.6. Ageism

Albeit sometimes used inappropriately in the existing literature, the term "ageism" means a prejudice, stereotyped assumption, or discrimination made on the grounds of a person's age, possibly leading to unfair treatment of older ones. From a clinical standpoint, an ageist attitude may lead clinicians to consider older adults' suicides as rational choices (especially if the person has physical illnesses) and affect clinicians' ability to identify psychopathology [54]. For instance, depression may seem understandable in the context of an older person's health and living circumstances, but considering suicidal ideation and wishes to die as understandable just because of the person's old age is an ageist attitude which should be avoided. Nonetheless, some studies [32] have pointed out that while clinicians' skills in identifying suicidal behaviour in older adults seem to be preserved, what may be lacking is their willingness to treat patients in this age group, especially if the potential reversibility of their condition is underestimated. This attitude too may reflect ageism and therapeutic nihilism. On the other hand, the implementation of coercive life-prolonging measures with a poor consideration of the individual's autonomy is another potential form of ageism hidden behind medical paternalism [36].

Trying to find a balance between patients' autonomy and clinicians' responsibility, therapeutic nihilism and medical paternalism is necessary to face a phenomenon, which may be associated with increased longevity.

3.7. Slippery Slope

Several authors have expressed concern that recognizing the right to die would too easily shift to "a climate enforcing a social, obligatory duty to die", and novelists have well described this risk in science fiction stories such us Richard Matheson's The Test (1958).

Indeed, several of the selected papers mentioned the "slippery slope" argument, which is also debated in the end-of-life/euthanasia/PAS/PAD context and which refers to the possibility that acknowledging the right to die would eventually shift towards an obligation to die and/or lead older persons to feel guilty if they had no wish to end their life and decided not to commit suicide [21].

However, it has to be underscored that, in the context of the euthanasia debate, no consensus has yet been reached about the presence of the slippery slope effect [64,65].

4. Discussion

The aim of this review was to offer an overview and a better understanding of the concept of rational suicide in older adults.

Opinions are not consistent about whether older adults' wish to hasten death in the absence of a psychiatric disorder could be regarded as a rational choice. Suicide presenting in the absence of a clinically diagnosable depression (or of other conditions impairing mental function) and occurring in cases of adverse conditions such as physical illness and aging has been considered "rational" from the perspective of respect for individual autonomy, and the rational assessment of utility [52]. Suicide in these situations may be seen as a possibility to regain and exert control and autonomy in the face of a miserable existential condition marked by pain and suffering, before the progressive worsening of one's physical condition, thus finding an escape from a life which is no longer considered as such or worth living.

Even though Authors do not agree on the role of mental disorders in "rational suicide", usually those who adhere to the conventional psychiatric opinion think that mental disorders are preeminent with regard to suicidal ideation and that suicide is a manifestation of psychiatric illness, hence they do not consider suicide as a rational option [40,54]. The possibility to disentangle depression and suicidal ideation in old-age suicidal individuals would allow the identification of potential targets for ad hoc interventions, going beyond those specifically directed towards the treatment of depression. For instance, there might still be chances, even for terminally ill and/or disabled older adults, to find relief from their pain and suffering, which could eventually lead to a decrease in suicidal ideation and suicide risk [19]. Furthermore, the perspective considering suicide as a symptom of psychiatric illness overlooks the possibility that there may be circumstances in which suicide or the refusal of life-sustaining medical treatment may result from the rational decisions of autonomous individuals, and may lead to interventions aimed at preserving life which can sometimes be applied at the expense of individual autonomy[40].

Although life expectancy for those living in western societies is higher than ever before in human history, this has had the effect of making it difficult for medical professionals to find a balance between patients' autonomy and clinicians' responsibility, to admit when someone is dying and to know where to draw the line in terms of offering more treatment [66,67]. The improvement of late life palliative care and QoL should be possibly accompanied by changes in the medical organization and culture to better address the specific end of life related needs in old age.

Some valuable suggestions to face the problem of rational suicide emerge from the studies we assessed; for instance, Richman, quoted by Moore [44] underscored the primary importance, when meeting a suicidal individual, "to make contact rather than obsess over whether they have a right to live or die". The importance of an interlocutory and reflective attitude is described by Ruckenbauer and coworkers [48], who state that while suicidal individuals cannot be deprived of their autonomy, nonetheless they should not be fully and without protection be released into their autonomy. Moreover, they underscore that patients cannot be reduced to their medical or psychiatric illness, but at the same time, an overestimation of existential stock-taking should be avoided.

It should be underscored that a limitation of this work is that, since the available literature was very uneven and, despite the selection criteria, mainly based on opinions and theoretical papers, the reported quantitative synthesis is limited. Furthermore, we cannot exclude that the choice of not including editorials and book chapters in the current review might have limited the access to potentially relevant material. Further original research studies may help to better understand this complex topic.

5. Conclusions

In conclusion, despite contrasting positions and inconsistencies of the studies described in this review, what seems to emerge is that the expression of suicidal thoughts in older adults, as well as behaviours suggesting "silent" or indirect suicidal attitudes [68,69], should be carefully investigated and addressed, even in the absence of a diagnosable mental disorder. Clinicians should try to decode the possible communicative role of suicidal behaviour while avoiding premature conclusions about the "rationality" of patients' decision to die, and considering it by default as "reasoned behavioural expression of legitimate preference for an earlier death" [7,46,49,70]. Nonetheless, the possibility of rational suicide cannot be precluded.

Author Contributions: Each author made substantial contributions to the conception and design of the work; C.G. and R.C. searched the literature and read the papers, under the supervision of P.Z.; C.G. and R.C. drafted the paper and P.Z. revised it; AND each author has approved the submitted version; AND agrees to be personally accountable for the author's own contributions and for ensuring that questions related to the accuracy or integrity of any part of the work, even ones in which the author was not personally involved, are appropriately investigated, resolved, and documented in the literature.

Funding: This research received no external funding.

Conflicts of Interest: The authors declare no conflicts of interest.

References

1. WHO. Suicide in the Western Pacific. Available online: https://www.who.int/westernpacific/health-topics/suicide (accessed on 16 August 2019).
2. Cheung, G.; Douwes, G.; Sundram, F. Late-Life Suicide in Terminal Cancer: A Rational Act or Underdiagnosed Depression? *J. Pain Symptom Manag.* **2017**, *54*, 835–842. [CrossRef] [PubMed]
3. Conwell, Y.; Thompson, C. Suicidal behavior in elders. *Psychiatr. Clin. N. Am.* **2008**, *31*, 333–356. [CrossRef] [PubMed]
4. Zeppegno, P.; Manzetti, E.; Valsesia, R.; Siliquini, R.; Ammirata, G.; De Donatis, O.; Usai, C.; Torre, E. Differences in suicide behaviour in the elderly: A study in two provinces of Northern Italy. *Int. J. Geriatr. Psychiatry* **2005**, *20*, 769–775. [CrossRef]

5. Institute of Medicine (US) Committee on Pathophysiology and Prevention of Adolescent and Adult Suicide. *Reducing Suicide: A National Imperative*; Goldsmith, S.K., Pellmar, T.C., Kleinman, A.M., Bunney, W.E., Eds.; National Academies Press (US): Washington, DC, USA, 2002. Available online: http://www.ncbi.nlm.nih.gov/books/NBK220939/ (accessed on 16 August 2019).
6. Zeppegno, P.; Gramaglia, C.; di Marco, S.; Guerriero, C.; Consol, C.; Loreti, L.; Martelli, M.; Marangon, D.; Carli, V.; Sarchiapone, M. Intimate Partner Homicide Suicide: A Mini-Review of the Literature (2012–2018). *Curr. Psychiatry Rep.* **2019**, *21*, 13. [CrossRef] [PubMed]
7. Simon, R.I. Silent suicide in the elderly. *Bull. Am. Acad. Psychiatry Law* **1989**, *17*, 83–95.
8. Conwell, Y.; Duberstein, P.R.; Cox, C.; Herrmann, J.H.; Forbes, N.T.; Caine, E.D. Relationships of age and axis I diagnoses in victims of completed suicide: A psychological autopsy study. *Am. J. Psychiatry* **1996**, *153*, 1001–1008.
9. Turvey, C.L.; Conwell, Y.; Jones, M.P.; Phillips, C.; Simonsick, E.; Pearson, J.L.; Wallace, R. Risk factors for late-life suicide: A prospective, community-based study. *Am. J. Geriatr. Psychiatry* **2002**, *10*, 398–406. [CrossRef] [PubMed]
10. Sokero, T.P.; Melartin, T.K.; Rytsälä, H.J.; Leskelä, U.S.; Lestelä-Mielonen, P.S.; Isometsä, E.T. Suicidal ideation and attempts among psychiatric patients with major depressive disorder. *J. Clin. Psychiatry* **2003**, *64*, 1094–1100. [CrossRef] [PubMed]
11. Fässberg, M.M.; Cheung, G.; Canetto, S.S.; Erlangsen, A.; Lapierre, S.; Lindner, R.; Draper, B.; Gallo, J.J.; Wong, C.; Wu, J.; et al. A systematic review of physical illness, functional disability, and suicidal behaviour among older adults. *Aging Ment. Health* **2016**, *20*, 166–194. [CrossRef] [PubMed]
12. Rurup, M.L.; Pasman, H.R.W.; Goedhart, J.; Deeg, D.J.H.; Kerkhof, A.J.F.M.; Onwuteaka-Philipsen, B.D. Understanding why older people develop a wish to die: A qualitative interview study. *Crisis* **2011**, *32*, 204–216. [CrossRef]
13. Balasubramaniam, M. Rational Suicide in Elderly Adults: A Clinician's Perspective. *J. Am. Geriatr. Soc.* **2018**, *66*, 998–1001. [CrossRef] [PubMed]
14. Erikson, E.H. *Childhood and Society*; WW Norton & Company: New York, NY, USA, 1993.
15. Muskin, P.R. The request to die: Role for a psychodynamic perspective on physician-assisted suicide. *JAMA* **1998**, *279*, 323–328. [CrossRef] [PubMed]
16. Arie, T. On Aging. In *Revolt and Resignation*; Jean Amery; Indiana University Press: Bloomington, IN, USA, 1994; p. 132.
17. Siegel, K. Psychosocial aspects of rational suicide. *Am. J. Psychother.* **1986**, *40*, 405–418. [CrossRef]
18. Mayo, D.J. The concept of rational suicide. *J. Med. Philos.* **1986**, *11*, 143–155. [CrossRef] [PubMed]
19. Valente, S.M.; Trainor, D. Rational suicide among patients who are terminally ill. *AORN J.* **1998**, *68*, 252–258, 260–264. [CrossRef]
20. Moody, H.R. *Ethics in an Aging Society*; Johns Hopkins University Press Books: Baltimore, MD, USA, 1992; Volume 1, Available online: https://jhupbooks.press.jhu.edu/title/ethics-aging-society (accessed on 17 August 2019).
21. Siegel, K. Rational suicide: Considerations for the clinician. *Psychiatr. Q.* **1982**, *54*, 77–84. [CrossRef]
22. Werth, J.L.; Cobia, D.C. Empirically based criteria for rational suicide: A survey of psychotherapists. *Suicide Life Threat. Behav.* **1995**, *25*, 231–240. [PubMed]
23. Motto, J.A. The Right to Suicide: A Psychiatrist's View. *Suicide Life Threat. Behav.* **1972**, *2*, 183–188.
24. Diekstra, R.F.W. The significance of Nico Speiler's suicide: How and when should suicide be prevented? *Suicide Life Threat. Behav.* **1986**, *16*, 13–15. [CrossRef]
25. Humphry, D. Rational suicide among the elderly. *Suicide Life Threat. Behav.* **1992**, *22*, 125–129.
26. A Cliff, Not a Slope: A Response to Margaret P. Battin. Centre for Suicide Prevention. Available online: https://www.suicideinfo.ca/resource/siecno-19890235/ (accessed on 17 August 2019).
27. Graber, G.C. The rationality of suicide. In *Suicide and Euthanasia: The Rights of Personhood*, 1st ed.; Wallace, S.E., Eser, A., Eds.; University of Tennessee Press: Knoxville, TN, USA, 1981; pp. 51–65.
28. Rich, K.L.; Butts, J.B. Rational suicide: Uncertain moral ground. *J. Adv. Nurs.* **2004**, *46*, 270–278. [CrossRef] [PubMed]
29. Moher, D. Preferred Reporting Items for Systematic Reviews and Meta-Analyses: The PRISMA Statement. *Ann. Intern. Med.* **2009**, *151*, 264. [CrossRef] [PubMed]

30. Fortin, A.; Lapierre, S.; Baillargeon, J.; Labelle, R.; Dubé, M.; Pronovost, J. Suicidal ideation and self-determination in institutionalized elderly. *Crisis* **2001**, *22*, 15–19. [CrossRef] [PubMed]
31. Gibbs, L.M.; Dombrovski, A.Y.; Morse, J.; Siegle, G.J.; Houck, P.R.; Szanto, K. When the solution is part of the problem: Problem solving in elderly suicide attempters. *Int. J. Geriatr. Psychiatry* **2009**, *24*, 1396–1404. [CrossRef]
32. Uncapher, H.; Areán, P.A. Physicians are less willing to treat suicidal ideation in older patients. *J. Am. Geriatr. Soc.* **2000**, *48*, 188–192. [CrossRef]
33. Van Wijngaarden, E.; Leget, C.; Goossensen, A. Caught between intending and doing: Older people ideating on a self-chosen death. *BMJ Open* **2016**, *6*, e009895. [CrossRef]
34. Winterrowd, E.; Canetto, S.S.; Benoit, K. Permissive beliefs and attitudes about older adult suicide: A suicide enabling script? *Aging Ment. Health* **2017**, *21*, 173–181. [CrossRef]
35. Lerner, B.H. Knowing when to say goodbye: Final Exit and suicide in the elderly. *Suicide Life Threat. Behav.* **1995**, *25*, 508–512.
36. Wand, A.P.F.; Peisah, C.; Draper, B.; Jones, C.; Brodaty, H. Rational Suicide, Euthanasia, and the Very Old: Two Case Reports. *Case Rep. Psychiatry* **2016**, *2016*, 4242064. [CrossRef]
37. Battin, M.B. The Concept of Rational Suicide. 1984. Available online: https://scholar.google.com/scholar_lookup?title=The+concept+of+rational+suicide&author=M.+P.+Battin&publication_year=1984 (accessed on 16 August 2019).
38. Conwell, Y.; Caine, E.D. Rational suicide and the right to die. Reality and myth. *N. Engl. J. Med.* **1991**, *325*, 1100–1103. [CrossRef]
39. Fontana, J.S. Rational suicide in the terminally ill. *J. Nurs. Scholarsh.* **2002**, *34*, 147–151. [CrossRef] [PubMed]
40. Karlinsky, H.; Taerk, G.; Schwartz, K.; Ennis, J.; Rodin, G. Suicide attempts and resuscitation dilemmas. *Gen. Hosp. Psychiatry* **1988**, *10*, 423–430. [CrossRef]
41. Werth, J.L. *Contemporary Perspectives on Rational Suicide [Internet]*; Brunner/Mazel: Philadelphia, PA, USA, 1999. Available online: https://trove.nla.gov.au/work/8768140 (accessed on 16 April 2019).
42. Gallagher-Thompson, D.; Osgood, N.J. Suicide in later life. *Behav. Ther.* **1997**, *28*, 23–41. [CrossRef]
43. Battin, M.P. Rational suicide: How can we respond to a request for help? *Crisis* **1991**, *12*, 73–80.
44. Moore, S.L. Rational suicide among older adults: A cause for concern? *Arch. Psychiatr. Nurs.* **1993**, *7*, 106–110. [CrossRef]
45. Prado, C.G. Ageism and elective death. *Ethics Med. Public Health* **2015**, *1*, 442–449. [CrossRef]
46. Richards, N. Old age rational suicide. *Sociol. Compass* **2017**, *11*, e12456. [CrossRef]
47. McCue, R.; Balasubramaniam, M. *Rational Suicide in the Elderly—Clinical, Ethical, and Sociocultural Aspects*; Springer Ebooks: New York, NY, USA, 2017; Available online: https://www.springer.com/gp/book/9783319326702 (accessed on 16 August 2019).
48. Ruckenbauer, G.; Yazdani, F.; Ravaglia, G. Suicide in old age: Illness or autonomous decision of the will? *Arch. Gerontol. Geriatr.* **2007**, *44* (Suppl. 1), 355–358. [CrossRef]
49. Clark, D.C. "Rational" suicide and people with terminal conditions or disabilities. *Issues Law Med.* **1992**, *8*, 147–166. [PubMed]
50. Den Hartogh, G. Two Kinds of Suicide. *Bioethics* **2016**, *30*, 672–680. [CrossRef]
51. Torre, E.; Zeppegno, P.; Usai, C.; Rudoni, M.; Ammirata, G.; De Donatis, O.; Manzetti, E.; Marangon, D.; Migliaretti, G. Suicide in Verbano-Cusio-Ossola province: Decade 1990–2000. *Epidemiol. Psichiatr. Soc.* **2002**, *11*, 277–283. [CrossRef] [PubMed]
52. Clarke, D.M. Autonomy, rationality and the wish to die. *J. Med. Ethics* **1999**, *25*, 457–462. [CrossRef] [PubMed]
53. Maris, R. Rational Suicide: An Impoverished Self-Transformation. *Suicide Life Threat. Behav.* **1982**, *12*, 4–16. [CrossRef]
54. Richman, J. The Case against Rational Suicide. *Suicide Life Threat. Behav.* **1988**, *18*, 285–289. [CrossRef] [PubMed]
55. Shneidman, E.S. Psychotherapy with suicidal patients. *Suicide Life Threat. Behav.* **1981**, *11*, 341–348.
56. Stiefel, F.; Die Trill, M.; Berney, A.; Olarte, J.M.; Razavi, A. Depression in palliative care: A pragmatic report from the Expert Working Group of the European Association for Palliative Care. *Support. Care Cancer* **2001**, *9*, 477–488. [CrossRef] [PubMed]
57. Passik, S.D.; Dugan, W.; McDonald, M.V.; Rosenfeld, B.; Theobald, D.E.; Edgerton, S. Oncologists' recognition of depression in their patients with cancer. *J. Clin. Oncol.* **1998**, *16*, 1594–1600. [CrossRef] [PubMed]

58. McDonald, M.V.; Passik, S.D.; Dugan, W.; Rosenfeld, B.; Theobald, D.E.; Edgerton, S. Nurses' recognition of depression in their patients with cancer. *Oncol. Nurs. Forum* **1999**, *26*, 593–599. [PubMed]
59. Block, S.D. Assessing and managing depression in the terminally ill patient. ACP-ASIM End-of-Life Care Consensus Panel. American College of Physicians—American Society of Internal Medicine. *Ann. Intern. Med.* **2000**, *132*, 209–218. [CrossRef]
60. Periyakoil, V.S.; Kraemer, H.C.; Noda, A.; Moos, R.; Hallenbeck, J.; Webster, M.; Yesavage, J.A. The development and initial validation of the terminally illgreif of depression scale (TIGDS). *Int. J. Methods Psychiatr. Res.* **2005**, *14*, 202–212. [CrossRef] [PubMed]
61. Osgood, N.J. *Suicide in the Elderly. A Practitioner's Guide to Diagnosis and Mental Health Intervention*; Aspen Systems Corporation: Rockville, MD, USA, 1985.
62. Kerkhof, A.; de Leo, D. Suicide in the elderly: A frightful awareness. *Crisis* **1991**, *12*, 81–87. [PubMed]
63. Schneewind, E.H. Of ageism, suicide, and limiting life. *J. Gerontol. Soc. Work* **1994**, *23*, 135–150. [CrossRef]
64. Reggler, J. The slippery slope argument and medical assistance in dying. *CMAJ* **2017**, *189*, E471. [CrossRef] [PubMed]
65. Potter, J. The psychological slippery slope from physician-assisted death to active euthanasia: A paragon of fallacious reasoning. *Med. Health Care Philos.* **2019**, *22*, 239–244. [CrossRef]
66. Kaufman, S.R. *Ordinary Medicine: Extraordinary Treatments, Longer Lives, and Where to Draw the Line (Critical Global Health: Evidence, Efficacy, Ethnography)*; Duke University Press: Durham, NC, USA, 2015.
67. Gawande, A. *Being Mortal Illness, Medicine and What Matters in the End*; Profile Books Ltd.: London, UK, 2014.
68. Farberow, N.L. (Ed.) *The Many Faces of Suicide: Indirect Self-Destructive Behavior*; McGraw-Hill: New York, NY, USA, 1980.
69. Shneidman, E.S. *Deaths of Man*; Quadrangle: New York, NY, USA, 1973.
70. Conwell, Y.; Pearson, J.; De Renzo, E. Indirect self-destructive behavior among elderly patients in nursing homes: A research agenda. *Am. J. Geriatr. Psychiatry* **1996**, *4*, 152–163. [CrossRef] [PubMed]

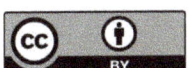

© 2019 by the authors. Licensee MDPI, Basel, Switzerland. This article is an open access article distributed under the terms and conditions of the Creative Commons Attribution (CC BY) license (http://creativecommons.org/licenses/by/4.0/).

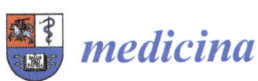

Review

The Meaning in Life in Suicidal Patients: The Presence and the Search for Constructs. A Systematic Review

Alessandra Costanza [1,2,*], Massimo Prelati [2] and Maurizio Pompili [3]

1. Department of Psychiatry, Faculty of Medicine, University of Geneva (UNIGE), 1206 Geneva, Switzerland
2. Department of Psychiatry, ASO Santi Antonio e Biagio e Cesare Arrigo Hospital, 15121 Alessandria, Italy
3. Department of Neurosciences, Mental Health and Sensory Organs, Suicide Prevention Center, Sant'Andrea Hospital, Sapienza University of Rome, 00185 Rome, Italy
* Correspondence: alessandra.costanza@unige.ch

Received: 13 June 2019; Accepted: 6 August 2019; Published: 11 August 2019

Abstract: *Background and Objectives:* Research on suicidal behavior (SB) has frequently focused more on risk factors than protective factors. Since the historic works of Viktor E. Frankl, who inquired how some Nazi concentration camps prisoners maintained their will to live though confronted with pervasive absurdity, Meaning in Life (MiL) has been interpreted as a potent resiliency factor. MiL then declined along a multitude of theoretical perspectives and was associated with various functioning domains of the individual. Surprising, few studies investigated the role of MiL on SB. We aimed to review and synthetize current literature on possible associations between MiL and SB, which included suicidal ideation (SI), suicidal attempts (SA), and completed suicide, focusing on two MiL constructs (the presence of MiL and search for MiL) from the Michael F. Steger's recent conceptualization. *Material and Methods:* A systematic strategy following PRISMA guidelines was used to search for relevant articles in Pubmed/MEDLINE, Scopus, PsycINFO, and ScienceDirect (January 1980–February 2019) and yielded 172 articles, 37 of which met our inclusion criteria. *Results:* MiL emerged as a protective factor against SI, SA, and completed suicides, directly or through mediation/moderation models with other SB-related variables. When distinguishing the presence of MiL and the search for MiL, a consensual protective impact was described for the former. Data for the latter were less consistent but rather oriented towards a non-protective impact *Conclusions:* These findings could have clinical repercussions for SB prevention, in both suicide risk assessment refinement and psychotherapeutic interventions. Further research is needed to examine the dynamic interplay of the two constructs.

Keywords: suicide; suicidal behavior; suicidal ideation; suicide attempt; meaning in life; suicide protective factors; suicide risk

1. Introduction

Research on suicidal behavior (SB) has frequently focused on suicide risk factors. In contrast, elements that can buffer stressors and protect an individual from SB have received less attention [1]. Historically, exploration into the adaptive and life-maintaining characteristics of non-suicidal people was originated by Viktor E. Frankl, who attempted to elucidate how some Nazi concentration camp prisoners were able to maintain the will to live and which subjective reasons protected them from a pervasive sense of absurdity [2]. He observed that individuals with a "will of meaning" (*Der Wille zum Sinn*) had the best chance of survival [2]. On this basis, Frankl elaborated the discovery path of Meaning in Life (MiL) against the "existential vacuum" as arising from three possible assumptions, uniquely concerning the human condition: (1) creativity (related to the sense of realization of an individual), (2) perception and a search for beauty (in relation to a sense of authenticity towards certain situations or encounters), and (3) the effort of an individual in trying to find a way to determine one's interior attitude, even when overwhelmed by miserable circumstances or unavoidable suffering [2].

Since Frankl's initial observations, Meaning in Life (MiL) has been described from a multitude of theoretical perspectives. One primary distinction has been made between a "global or existential" meaning and a "situational or specific" meaning, thereby discerning individuals' fundamental assumptions from meaning in the context of a particular environmental encounter [3–6]. In this latter area, the integrated model of "meaning-making", articulated by Crystal L. Park, is of particular interest [4]. In addition to the distinction between "global" and "situational" meaning, Park proposed the evaluation of "meaning-making efforts" and "meaning made", inscribing the possible effects of all these subconstructs in a meaning-making process aimed at adjusting one's experiences of events that are greatly discrepant with one's larger beliefs, plans, and desires [4].

In the recent psychological literature, Michael F. Steger has proposed that the greatest consensus in the conceptualization of MiL can be centered on two dimensions: "coherence", or a sense of the comprehensibility and self-concordant ability of making sense in one's life, and "purpose", or a sense of core goals, aims, and direction in life [7]. A third facet, "significance", which focuses on values, worth, and the importance of one's life, is receiving increasing attention [7]. "Coherence" refers to the cognitive component of MiL, focusing on the perception that stimuli are predictable and conform to recognizable personal patterns that transcend chaos. "Coherence" would be especially activated in situations where meaning is disrupted and the individual experiences distress and the related necessity to construct or reconstruct a framework to understand life [7]. While "purpose" is sometimes used synonymously with MiL, it should be explicitly considered separately from the general sense of MiL and understood as one of its components (the motivational one), based on one's goals and enthusiasm in life (e.g., spirituality and religiousness were shown to be correlated to MiL but not to "purpose", while optimism was correlated to "purpose" but not to MiL) [7]. "Significance" constitutes the evaluative component for MiL as it relates to how important, worthwhile, and inherently valuable one's life as a whole feels beyond trivial or momentary elements [7]. Both "purpose" and "significance" are value-laden concepts, but they differ in two essential aspects, based on their primary motivational versus evaluative nature. "Purpose" is about finding valuable goals future-oriented, while "significance" is about finding value in life, including the past, present, and future [7]. When all three components are taken together, a definition for MiL emerges from "the web of connections, interpretations, aspirations, and evaluations" that "(1) make our experiences comprehensible, (2) direct our efforts toward a desired future, and (3) provide a sense that our lives matter and are worthwhile" [7,8].

Steger's model divides MiL into two constructs: the presence of MiL and the search for MiL [9]. These two constructs were found not to be mutually exclusive [10]. The presence of MiL is uniformly thought to be beneficial for various functional aspects of life, including adaptive resources, overall psychological well-being, and positive affects [11]. By contrast, the search for MiL appears more controversial. Some researchers consider MiL the essence of human motivation [12,13], while others find it a dysfunctional sign that meaning has been frustrated or lost [14,15]. In a third perspective, the search for MiL can have either healthy or non-healthy connotations depending on the motivational [3] and personal characteristics of the individual [16]. Addressing this issue from a typological perspective, MiL profiles resulting from a combination of high scores in the presence of MiL and low scores in the search for MiL have been associated with better adjustment outcomes [17,18]. Both constructs are highly stable over time, suggesting that MiL more accurately reflects a trait aspect than a state aspect of individual functioning [18].

From a clinical viewpoint, exploring MiL in suicidal patients during psychiatric interviews would personalize and improve their SB risk assessments [19,20]. Interventions targeting MiL have also been found effective in reducing suicide risk [21] and represent a promising therapeutic opportunity [19,20,22].

Few studies have explored MiL in individuals presenting SB. With this review, we aimed to examine existing published data to investigate possible associations between MiL and suicidal ideation (SI), suicide attempts (SA), and completed suicide. Particular attention was given to studies that distinguished between the roles of the presence of MiL and the search for MiL. We hypothesized that MiL has a protective effect on SI, SA, and completed suicide. Specifically, for works that addressed the two constructs of MiL, we hypothesized that the presence of MiL would have a protective effect. The exiguity and contradictory nature of the data on the search for MiL did not allow us to formulate a specific hypothesis but only to perform exploratory analyses.

2. Methods

This review was conducted according to the Preferred Reporting Items for Systematic Reviews and Meta-Analyses (PRISMA) guidelines [23] and the Cochrane collaboration guidelines [24].

2.1. Information Sources and Search Strategy

We performed a systematic search in four major electronic databases comprising medical and social science research (PubMed/MEDLINE, Scopus, Science Direct, and PsychINFO) for relevant titles and abstracts published between January 1980 and February 2019. Additional articles were retrieved from the reference lists of relevant articles and from published reviews. The following combined search queries of free-text terms and exploded Medical Subject Headings (MeSH) terms were used for the Pubmed/MEDLINE database: "Meaning in Life" AND "Suicidal ideation" [MeSH] OR "Suicide, attempted" [MeSH] OR "Suicide" [MeSH] OR "Suicidal Behavior" OR "suicidality." This search strategy was adapted for use with the other databases.

2.2. Eligibility Criteria

Articles that explicitly mentioned a potential association between MiL and SB (OR suicidal ideation OR suicide attempts OR completed suicides) in non-clinical and clinical samples were included. When a title or abstract seemed to describe an eligible study, the full-text article was obtained and carefully examined to assess the study's relevance for our review. Our exclusion criteria were: (1) articles published before 1980, (2) articles with abstracts that did not directly mention an investigation into a potential association between MiL and SB, (3) articles not published in peer-reviewed journals, (4) articles not published in English, and (5) meta-analytic, systematic, or narrative reviews, or book chapters.

2.3. Study Selection and Data Collection

Studies were independently reviewed by two authors (A.C. and M.Pre.) using a two-step process. First, screening and selection were performed based on the article's title and abstract. Second, further screenings and selections were performed on retrieved full-text articles. A data extraction spreadsheet was developed [23]. The data were extracted by one author (A.C.) and supervised by another (M.Pre.). The data elements of interest were author(s), publication year, study design, sample characteristics (population type, sample size, and psychiatric diagnosis when appropriate), instrument(s) used to assess MiL, and the impact on SB-related variables (SI, SA, completed suicide, other SB-related variables, and/or main commentaries). At any stage of the article selection and data collection processes, disagreements were resolved through discussion with the senior reviewer (M.Pom.), who also independently read all the articles.

2.4. Summary Measures

As with previous studies [25,26], we assessed the selected studies for quality using the following criteria: (1) the representativeness of the sample for the general population, (2) the presence and representativeness of a control group, (3) the presence of longitudinal follow-up, (4) the evidence-based measures of MiL (e.g., a Meaning in Life Questionnaire, Purpose in Life Questionnaire, or other psychometric instruments), (5) the presence of raters who independently identified MiL, (6) the statistical evaluation of inter-rater reliability, and (7) evidence-based measures of SI or SA (e.g., a Suicidal Ideation Questionnaire, Suicide Risk Scale, Beck Hopelessness Scale, or other psychometric evaluation). A score of 0–2 points was attributed to each item, yielding a quality score ranging from 0 to 14. Studies were divided into 3 groups: (1) good quality (10–14 points), if most or all the criteria were fulfilled, or, where they were not met, the study conclusions were deemed very robust; (2) moderate quality (5–9 points), if some criteria were fulfilled or the study conclusions were deemed robust; or (3) low quality (0–4 points), if few criteria were fulfilled or the study conclusions were not deemed robust. Caution was adopted in interpreting the findings from the low-quality studies. Disagreements between reviewers were resolved by consensus.

3. Results

3.1. Included Studies

After removing 61 duplicates, a total of 172 potentially relevant articles were found. Figure 1 shows the flow through the identification, screening, and assessment of eligibility. Studies were excluded either because the exclusion criteria were met or because of low relevance compared to our primary theme. Finally, 37 studies met our inclusion criteria and were included in our qualitative synthesis for this review.

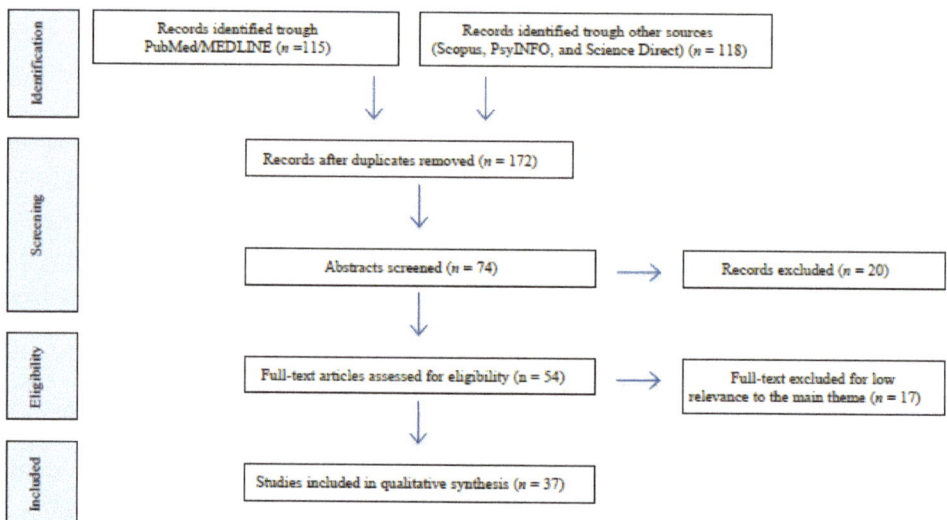

Figure 1. Flowchart for the search and selection process [23].

3.2. Characteristics of Included Studies (Study Designs and Samples)

The characteristics of the included studies are shown in Tables 1 and 2. In total, 24 studies were cross-sectional, nine were prospective and longitudinal, and five were qualitative (one was classified as both cross-sectional and longitudinal). Additionally, 20 were conducted using non-clinical populations (Tables 1 and 2), and 17 were conducted using psychiatric and non-psychiatric clinical populations (Tables 1 and 2). Among the non-clinical populations, undergraduate students and adolescents were the most frequently represented groups ($n = 12$) followed by elderly people ($n = 7$). Eight studies included individuals aged 12–70 years, one included only adults, and one included individuals aged at least 20 years and was based on the general population participating in the Nord-Trøndelag Health Study in Norway (the HUNT I cohort during 1984–1986 and the HUNT II cohort during 1995–1997). The specific studied populations were military personnel and veterans ($n = 3$), Chinese professional employees ($n = 1$), homeless people ($n = 1$), and disadvantaged African American female survivors of a recent SA ($n = 1$). Among studies performed using clinical populations, mood disorders were the most specifically addressed psychiatric diagnoses ($n = 6$), followed by borderline personality disorders ($n = 3$). Finally, five studies were performed based on various mental disorders (including mood and anxiety disorders, borderline and avoidant personality disorder, and post-traumatic stress disorder (PTSD), eating disorders, substance use disorder, and psychotic spectrum disorder), two were based on PTSD alone, and one was based on eating disorders. The only clinical non-psychiatric population studied was the population diagnosed as HIV-positive.

Of the studies that addressed the impact of the two MiL-distinct constructs (the presence of MiL and the search for MiL) ($n = 5$; Table 2), one was both cross-sectional and prospective, two were cross-sectional, and two were longitudinal and prospective. No qualitative studies were represented in this group. Three studies were conducted among non-clinical populations (two among undergraduate students and one among soldiers returning from deployment; Table 2), and two were conducted among clinical populations (one among patientss diagnosed with severe PTSD/depression and one among those diagnosed as HIV-positive; Table 2).

Interest in this research subject has increased over very recent years (32 of the included studies were published in 2013 or later). This was particularly evident among studies conducted using clinical populations (12 of these 17 studies were published in 2015 or later). Most of these ($n = 7$) were performed using Spanish clinical samples by Marco and colleagues. Of those performed using non-clinical samples of adolescents/undergraduate students, nearly half (5 of 12) were performed using Israeli samples, and four of these were performed by Wilchek-Aviad and colleagues. Notably, all the studies that focused on the impact of the two MiL-distinct constructs (presence of MiL and search for MiL) were published in 2013 or later, and all but one were published in 2016 or later. Notably, two of the three studies using samples of military personnel and veterans focused on these two constructs.

Table 1. Studies investigating associations between meaning in life (MiL) and suicidal behavior (SB)-related variables ($N = 32$).

Non-Clinical Populations ($n = 17$)

Author(s)	Study Design	Sample Population	Size (N)	Instrument Assessing MiL	SI	SA	Completed Suicide	SB-Related Variables Other SB-Related Variables and/or Main Commentaries
Edwards and Holden, 2001 [27]	Cross-sectional	Undergraduate students	298	PIL, Sense of Coherence Scale	↓	↓	—	↓ Self-reported likelihood of future SB
Orbach et al., 2003 (study 2) [28]	Cross-sectional	Undergraduate students	98	LRI	—	—	—	MiL inversely related to mental pain
Wang et al., 2007 [1]	Cross-sectional	Undergraduate students	416	PIL	↓	↓	—	Mediation model: MiL mediated relationships between stress, coping, SI, and SA indirectly via an inverse effect on depression
Heisel and Flett, 2008 [29]	Cross-sectional	Elderly	107	GSIS Perceived MiL subscale	↓	—	—	—
Bjerkeset et al., 2010 [30]	Longitudinal prospective	Individuals aged 20+ yr, based on the Norwegian HUNT general population cohort	141,117	Self-reported measure of sense of MiL (n.sp.)	n.sp.	n.sp.	↓	A lower sense of MiL associated with increased suicide risk after controlling for common mental disorders that emerged during the survey
Kleiman et al., 2013 [31]	Longitudinal prospective	Undergraduate students	209	MLQ	↓	—	—	Mediated moderation model: gratitude and grit work synergistically to enhance MiL and confer resiliency to suicide by increasing MiL
Henry et al., 2014 [32]	Cross-sectional	Undergraduate students	2936	3-item MLQ	↓	—	—	Mediation model (female population): MiL could explain how bullying victimization leads to SI; moderation model (male population): effect of victimization on SI was attenuated as MiL increased
Wilchek-Aviad, 2015 [33]	Cross-sectional	Adolescents (Ethiopian immigrant and native-born Israeli)	277	PIL	—	—	—	↓ Suicidal tendencies (measured while accounting for depression and anxiety/emotional state) beyond one's immigrant and native-born status
Denneson et al., 2015 [22]	Qualitative	Veterans	34	Semi-structured interviews	↓	—	—	—
Heisel and Flett, 2016 [34]	Longitudinal prospective	Elderly	126	EMIL, PIL	↓	—	—	—

Table 1. Cont.

Non-Clinical Populations (n = 17)

Author(s)	Study Design	Sample Population	Size (N)	Instrument Assessing MiL	SI	SA	Completed Suicide	Other SB-Related Variables and/or Main Commentaries
Heisel et al., 2016 [35]	Longitudinal prospective	Elderly	109	EMIL	↓	—	—	Mediation model: MiL mediated associations between "Reasons for Living" and SI; it also explained the significant unique variance in SI
Wilchek-Aviad and Malka, 2016 [36]	Cross-sectional	Adolescents (Jewish religious and secular)	450	PIL	—	—	—	↓ Suicidal tendency (see above) beyond religiosity
Wilchek-Aviad et al., 2017 [37]	Cross-sectional	Adolescents (having different types of leisure time activities)	450	PIL	↓	—	—	MiL was greatest among adolescents involved in social endeavors, lower among those involved in solitary activities, and lowest among those not involved in any leisure activity
Wilchek-Aviad and Ne'eman-Haviv, 2018 [38]	Cross-sectional	Adolescent girls (disadvantaged at different stages of rehabilitation and normative)	209	PIL	—	—	—	↓ Suicidal potential (equivalent to the suicidal tendency, see above) among normative and disadvantaged adolescent girls residing in boarding schools
Schnell et al., 2018 [39]	Cross-sectional	Undergraduate students	300	Crisis of Meaning Scale	↓	↓	—	Crisis of meaning was distinguished from depression and predicted suicidality in youth independent of depression
Liu et al., 2018 [40]	Cross-sectional	Chinese professional employees	687	MLM	↓	—	—	Mediation model: MiL mediated relationships between psychological strain and SI
Testoni et al., 2018 [41]	Qualitative	Homeless people	55	Thematic and interpretative phenomenological analysis	↓	—	—	MiL was the most important reason for living; when it was considered unworkable, addiction/alcoholism represented a strategy to endure life in the street. Neither religiosity nor meaning of death were protective factors for addiction/alcoholism or SI

(A)

Table 1. Cont.

Author(s)	Study Design	Population	Sample Size (N)	Psychiatric Diagnosis	Instrument Assessing MiL	SI	SA	Completed Suicide	Other SB-Related Variables and Main Commentaries
Moore, 1997 [42]	Qualitative	Elderly	11	Depression	Hermeneutic analysis	↓	–	–	MiL descriptions were always tied to relational contexts: meaninglessness relative to missing (or perceived to be missing) connectedness
Heisel and Flett, 2004 [43]	Cross-sectional	Adults	49	Various	PIL	↓	–	–	MiL accounted for significant variance in SI—also, a mediation model between satisfaction in life and SI and a moderation model between depression and SI
van Orden et al., 2012 [44]	Longitudinal prospective	Elderly	65	Depression, anxiety	GSIS Perceived MiL subscale	–	–	–	"Perceived burdensomeness" might contribute to suicide morbidity and mortality by eroding MiL
Holm et al., 2014 [45]	Qualitative	Elderly	9	Mood disorder	Hermeneutic analysis	↓	–	–	MiL in the experience of SI was associated with existential aloneness: "Being alone without MiL"
Garcia-Alandete et al., 2014 [46]	Cross-sectional	16–60 yr old	80	Borderline personality disorder	PIL-10	–	–	–	↓ Suicide risk (measured accounting for general suicide risk factors),↓ depression,↓ hopelessness
van Orden et al., 2015 [47]	Qualitative	Elderly	101	Various	Semi-structured interviews	–	–	–	"Thwarted belongingness" was associated with more lethal methods and increased re-attempts
Braden et al., 2015 [48]	Cross-sectional	Veterans	110	Depressive disorder	LRI Framework subscale	↓	–	–	The relationship between MiL and SI remained significant after accounting for depressive symptoms, past SA, prior inpatient psychiatric hospitalization, and poor physical health
Marco et al., 2016 [19]	Cross-sectional	13–68 yr old	224	Various	PIL-10	–	–	–	Moderation model: MiL buffered associations between suicide risk factors and hopelessness
Marco et al., 2017a (study 2) [20]	Cross-sectional	13–70 yr old	80	Borderline personality disorder	PIL-10	–	→	–	MiL was also negatively correlated with other behavioral symptoms of borderline personality disorders, including suicidal threats, high-risk behaviors, drug overdoses, and aggressive behavior

Table 1. Cont.

Author(s)	Study Design	Population	Sample Size (N)	Psychiatric Diagnosis	Instrument Assessing MiL	SI	SA	Completed Suicide	SB-Related Variables Other SB-Related Variables and Main Commentaries
Marco et al., 2017b [49]	Cross-sectional	13–56 yr old	124	Borderline personality disorder	PIL-10	–	–	–	Moderation model: MiL buffered associations between suicide risk factors and hopelessness
Marco et al., 2017c [50]	Cross-sectional case-control	12–60 yr old	474	Eating disorder	PIL	↓	–	–	Patients with eating disorders had lower MiLs and greater SI than the controls; MiL predicts greater levels of both eating disorder psychopathologies and SI
Pérez Rodríguez et al., 2017a [51]	Cross-sectional	18–60 yr old	150	Various	PIL-10	–	NS	–	Hopelessness (specifically its affective component) differentiated between patients with non-suicidal self-injuries and those with SA but not MiL, which underlies the continuum of self-harm
Pérez Rodríguez et al., 2017b [52]	Cross-sectional	12–60 yr old	348	Various (mainly eating disorder)	PIL-10	–	↑	–	Lower levels of MiL and higher levels of hopelessness, borderline symptoms, and non-suicidal self-injuries were associated with SA in the previous year
Lamis et al., 2018 [53]	Cross-sectional	19–65 yr old	112	Bipolar disorder	SWBS (EWB + RWB)	↓	–	–	Existential MiL but not religious well-being acted as a protective factor against SI among bipolar disorder patients and those who experienced childhood sexual abuse
Florez et al., 2018 [54]	Longitudinal prospective	Disadvantaged African American female survivors of a recent SA	113	PTSD	SWBS (EWB + RWB)	↓	–	–	Mediation model: existential MiL, but not religious well-being, mediated the relationship between PTSD severity and both hopelessness and SI level

(B)

Note: MiL = Meaning in Life; SB = suicidal behavior; SI = suicidal ideation; SA = suicide attempt; PIL = Purpose in Life test; LRI = Life Regard Index; GSIS = Geriatric Suicide Ideation Scale; n.sp. = not specified; MLQ = Meaning in Life Questionnaire; 3-item MLQ = 3-item shortened version of the MLQ; EMIL = Experienced Meaning in Life instrument; PIL-10 = 10-item shortened version of the PIL; MLM = Meaningful Life Measure; yr = years; NS = not significant; SWBS = Spiritual Well-Being Scale; EWB = Existential Well-Being subscale; RWB = Religious Well-Being subscale.

Table 2. Studies investigating the associations between the the presence of MiL and the search for MiL and SB-related variables (N = 5).

(A) Non-Clinical Populations (n = 3)

Author(s)	Study Design	Sample Population	Sample Size (N)	Instrument Assessing MiL	SB-Related Variable: SI	SB-Related Variable: SA	SB-Related Variable: Completed Suicide	Other SB-Related Variables and/or Main Commentaries
Kleiman and Beaver, 2013 [55]	Cross-sectional and longitudinal prospective	Undergraduate students	670 (cross-sectional analysis); 585 (prospective analysis)	MLQ	↓ SI over time for both presence of MiL and search for MiL (greater effect for presence of MiL; minor effect for search for MiL)	↓ lifetime SA odds for presence of MiL	—	Additional findings: The presence of MiL, but not the search for MiL, mediated the relationship between MiL and the burdensomeness or thwarted belongingness and SI
Kim et al., 2017 [56]	Longitudinal prospective	Soldiers returning from deployment	970	MLQ	↓ for presence of MiL(miao) and ↑ for search for MiL	↓ for presence of MiL and(miao) ↑ for search for MiL	—	Suicide risk (including four dimensions of SI and SB): ↑ for the search for MiL; (miao)↓ for the presence of MiL (the latter was described by the authors as consistent but not significant)
Collins et al., 2018 [57]	Cross-sectional	Undergraduate students	93	MLQ (the presence of MiL subscal only)	—	—	—	An experimentally-enhanced presence conferred resilience to the interpersonal adversity ("perceived burdensomeness" or "thwarted belongingness") implicated in suicide risk

(B) Clinical Populations (n = 2)

Author(s)	Study Design	Sample Population	Sample Size (N)	Psychiatric Diagnosis	Instrument Assessing MiL	SB-Related Variables: SI	SB-Related Variables: SA	SB-Related Variables: Completed Suicide	Other SB-Related Variables and/or Main Commentaries
Sinclair et al., 2016 [58]	Cross-sectional	Military personnel and veterans	393	Elevated PTSD and depression	MLQ	—	—	—	Mediation model: The presence of MiL, but not search for MiL negatively mediated the relationship between PTSD or depression and the trajectory from SI to SA
Lu et al., 2018 [59]	Longitudinal prospective	HIV-positive patients	113	—	MLQ	↓ for presence of MiL, NS search for MiL	NS for presence of MiL; NS for search for MiL	—	Moderation model: The presence of MiL buffered the relationship between depressive symptoms and SI (no moderating effect between depressive symptoms and SA)

Note: MiL = Meaning in life; SB = suicidal behavior; SI = suicidal ideation; SA = suicide attempt; MLQ = Meaning in Life Questionnaire; PTSD = post-traumatic stress disorder; NS = not significant.

3.3. Quality Assessments

Based on our quality scoring system, the mean score of the included studies was 7.2. Most ($n = 16$) were of moderate quality, followed by those of low quality ($n = 14$) and those of good quality ($n = 7$).

3.4. Primary Findings

3.4.1. Studies of Associations between MiL and SB-Related Variables

The primary findings of the included studies that aimed to elucidate associations between MiL and SB-related variables are shown in Table 1. In these studies, MiL was assessed using either the Purpose in Life test [60] or its 10-item shortened version [61], the Geriatric Suicide Ideation Scale, the Perceived MiL subscale [62], the Experienced Meaning in Life instrument [63], the Life Regard Index [64,65], the Sense of Coherence Scale [66], the Crisis of Meaning Scale [67], the Meaningful Life Measure [68], the Spiritual Well-Being Scale (including the Existential Well-Being subscale and the Religious Well-Being subscale [69]), and qualitative analysis. Steger's Meaning in Life Questionnaire (MLQ) and its three-item shortened version [70] were also utilized, but without separate measures for the presence of, and search for, constructs.

Most studies investigated the impact of MiL on SI, and an inverse association was reported as direct [22,27,29,34,36,39,41–43,45,48,50,53] and/or through mediation and moderation models. MiL was found to mediate the relationships between SI and a variety of factors: stress/coping (via an inverse effect on depression) [1], "Reason for Living" [35], psychological strain [40], and satisfaction in life [43]. It was also found to mediate the relationship of both SI and hopelessness with PTSD severity [54]. Additionally, MiL was found to moderate associations between SI and depression [43] and between risk factors for suicide and hopelessness [19,49]. Both the mediation and moderation effects of MiL was found for gratitude and grit, which were shown to work synergistically to enhance MiL and confer resiliency to suicide by increasing MiL [31]. In bullying, a mediation model was reported in the female population, in which MiL explained how victimization can lead to SI, while a moderation model was reported in the male population, in which MiL attenuated the victimization effect on SI [32].

An inverse association between MiL and SA has been found in many studies [20,27,39,52]. Similar to the findings with SI, MiL was found to mediate the relationship between SA and stress/coping (via an inverse effect on depression) [1]. However, a moderation model was not described.

Only 1 study showed an inverse association between MiL and completed suicides. This result was based on two large cohorts of the general population [30]. The association remained significant after controlling for a common mental disorder that emerged during the survey. Unfortunately, only a published abstract was available for this study.

Inverse associations were also reported between MiL and suicidal tendency or suicidal potential (a measure accounting for depression, anxiety, and emotional state) [33,36,38] and between MiL and suicide risk (taking into account general suicide risk factors) [46].

Mental pain was inversely related to MiL [28] (study 2). Two variables of the Interpersonal-Psychology Theory of Suicide (IPTS) [71,72] were explored in relation to MiL. "Perceived burdensomeness" could contribute to suicide morbidity and mortality by eroding MiL [44], and "thwarted belongingness" was associated with more lethal methods for SA and increased SA [47]. Although not formally related to the IPTS, two additional context-relational variables were tied to meaninglessness in the SI experience: aloneness [45] and missing (or perceived missing) connectedness [42]. MiL, but neither religiosity [41] nor religious well-being [53,54], acted as protective factors against SI [41,53] and mediated the relationship between PTSD severity and both hopelessness and SI [54].

3.4.2. Studies of Associations between the Presence of MiL and the Search for MiL and SB-Related Variables

The primary findings of the included studies that aimed to elucidate associations between the presence of MiL and the search for MiL and SB-related variables are shown in Table 2. These two constructs of MiL were assessed using Steger's MLQ, which consists of a self-reported 10-item inventory measuring the extent to which individuals feel their lives are meaningful (the presence of MiL, five items) and the extent to which they are actively seeking meaning (the search for MiL, five items) [70].

Presence of MiL

The presence of MiL predicted decreased SI over time and lowered the lifetime odds of SA among undergraduate students in the longitudinal prospective analyses (with an average follow-up of 2 months) and cross-sectional analyses, respectively, from the same study [55]. These findings remained significant above and beyond the effects of low levels of psychopathology (depression and anxiety symptoms) and high levels of protective factors (gratitude and social support) [55]. In a study examining the factors related to changes in suicide risk among soldiers returning from deployment in Iraq and Afghanistan, surveyed 6 and 12 months following their return, the negative association between the presence of MiL and suicide risk became greater, but this finding was not statistically significant [56]. In this study, suicide risk was assessed using the Suicide Behavior Questionnaire-Revised, which includes four dimensions of SI and SB (lifetime SI and/or SA, frequency of SI over the past 12 months, the threat of SA, and self-reported likelihood of SB in the future) [73]. Among military personnel and veterans with severe PTSD and depression, the presence of MiL negatively mediated the relationship between PTSD or depression and the trajectory leading from the emergence of SI to SA [58]. The presence of MiL was found to moderate the association between depressive symptoms and SI but not the association between depressive symptoms and SA in HIV-positive patients 6 to 12 months following diagnosis [59]. Data for completed suicides were not available.

The presence of MiL mediated the relationships between MiL and the IPTS variables of "perceived burdensomeness" and "thwarted belongingness" and SI [55]. Additionally, the experimentally enhanced presence of MiL conferred resilience to perceived "burdensomeness and "thwarted belongingness" [57]. Both studies were performed using undergraduate students [55,57].

Search for MiL

The search for MiL predicted a decreased SI over time, but with a lower threshold for statistical significance than the presence of MiL, and it did not predict the lifetime odds of SA among undergraduate students [55]. In particular, the search for MiL was shown to predict post-deployment suicide risk, which increased among soldiers returning from deployment in Iraq and Afghanistan based on surveys administered 6 and 12 months following their return [56]. The strength of the association between initial depressive symptoms and becoming a high post-deployment suicide risk was diminished after accounting for the search for MiL. The search for MiL did not negatively mediate the relationship between PTSD or depression and the trajectory from SI to SA among military personnel and veterans [58]. Data for completed suicides were not available.

The search for MiL did not mediate the relationships between MiL and "perceived burdensomeness" or "thwarted belongingness" and SI [55], and it was not investigated in experimentally-enhanced conditions of interpersonal adversity [57] among undergraduate students [55,57].

4. Discussions

With this review, we have aimed to investigate the associations between MiL and SB, including SI, SA, and completed suicide. These associations have been examined in studies that considered MiL and those that distinguished the two MiL constructs (the presence of MiL and the search for MiL), according to Steger's model. We placed a particular focus on the latter.

The included studies consensually showed the protective impact of MiL on SI, SA, and completed suicide, whether conducted using clinical or non-clinical populations. In studies distinguishing the two MiL constructs (the presence of MiL and the search for MiL), a unanimous protective impact on SB-related variables was described only for the former. Correlations between the latter and SB-related variables were less consistent but were globally oriented towards a non-protective impact.

However, comparisons within the first group of studies are limited by an important heterogeneity in the neuropsychological assessment of MiL (Purpose in Life test, Geriatric Suicide Ideation Scale, Perceived MiL subscale, Experienced Meaning in Life instrument, Life Regard Index, Sense of Coherence Scale, Crisis of Meaning Scale, Meaningful Life Measure, Spiritual Well-Being Scale, and MLQ), presupposing different MiL conceptualizations that can overlap but cannot be considered synonymous [3,5,6]. By contrast, only one instrument, the MLQ [70], was utilized in the second group of studies, implying a more uniform MiL conceptualization upstream that includes the distinction between the presence of MiL and search for MiL.

Non-unanimous findings of the role of the search for MiL in SB reflect the debate surrounding the role of search for MiL in other functional aspects of individuals. In their longitudinal analysis of undergraduate students, Kleiman and Beaver [55] found that both the presence of MiL and the search for MiL predicted decreased SI over time, even if the statistical effect of the search for MiL was more marginal. Their cross-sectional analysis at baseline revealed, instead, that only the presence of MiL was associated with lower lifetime odds of SA. They argued that the search for MiL can only act as a protective factor against less severe manifestations of suicidality, which they supposed to be SI compared to SA. Their findings were especially interesting because the presence of MiL was shown to confer suicide resiliency independent of low levels of risk factors, such as psychopathology (depression and anxiety symptoms), and protective factors (gratitude and social support). However, they recognized a number of study limitations, which included the use of a non-clinical population, a large majority of female representatives in their sample, self-reporting of anxiety and depression symptoms, and a relatively small number of participants with a SA history, leading to an underpowered analysis based on SA [55].

The two studies performed using military personnel and veterans concluded only partially concordant findings on the beneficial versus deleterious impacts of the presence of MiL and search for MiL. Kim and colleagues [56] surveyed the suicide risk among soldiers returning from Iraq and Afghanistan twice during their first year post-deployment, observing that suicide risk increased significantly between the 6th and 12th months. Greater levels of search for MiL and perceived stress were associated with becoming a high suicide risk. The strength of the association between initial depressive symptoms and suicide risk was attenuated after accounting for these measures. On the other hand, they found a consistent negative association between the presence of MiL and becoming a high suicide risk post-deployment, but this relationship was not statistically significant [56]. The primary finding made by Sinclair and colleagues [58] in a study of military personnel and veterans with elevated levels of PTSD and depression was that the presence of MiL negatively mediated the relationship between PTSD or depression and the trajectory from SI to SA, particularly during acute experiences of mood disturbances. They estimated that this mediation was crucial for explaining why some military personnel and veterans do not become suicidal despite the correlation between their clinical conditions (PTSD/depression) and suicide risk. Contrary to their expectations, they found that search for MiL did not show the same mediation effect, suggesting that the active pursuit of MiL is not central to the trajectory from SI to SA [58].

In a clinical non-psychiatric cohort of HIV-positive patients surveyed 6 and 12 months after diagnosis (a population at high risk for both SI and SA), Lu and colleagues [59] reported that depressive symptoms were the primary predictors of changes in both SI and SA. Among the examined psychosocial factors, they found that only the presence of MiL buffered the relationship between depressive symptoms and SI. Neither the presence of MiL nor search for MiL showed a similar moderating effect on the relationship between depressive symptoms and SA [59].

Finally, Kleiman and Beaver [55] and Collins and colleagues [57] described the protective effect of the presence of MiL (but not the search for MiL) deployed on SI through two IPTS variables ("perceived burdensomeness" and "thwarted belongingness") described by Joiner and colleagues [71,72], in two cohorts of undergraduate students. According to IPTS, "perceived burdensomeness" and "thwarted belongingness" combine to produce SI [71,72]. The findings in the student samples mentioned above [55,57] were valorized because they potentially offered an additional way to explain and weaken the SI risk conferred by interpersonal adversities. However, both constructs were assessed in the former study [55], but only the presence of MiL was investigated (and manipulated in experimental conditions) in the latter study [57]. Inspired by IPTS, which marked a crucial turning point in suicide theories by distinguishing the emergence of SI from the progression from SI to SA (mediated in this case by the coexistence of a third variable, the "acquired suicidal capability"), another "Ideation-to-Action" framework was proposed by Klonsky and May: the Three-Step Theory of Suicide (3ST) [74]. This framework posits that SI first results from the combination of pain (usually psychological pain) and hopelessness. Second, among those experiencing both these conditions, connectedness is a key protective factor against SI escalation. Third, the progression from SI to SA is facilitated by dispositional, acquired, and practical contributors to the capacity to make SA [74]. In the theories of Joiners and colleagues and Klonsky and May, connectedness represents an essential resource and a fundamental step in the passage from suicidal ideation to suicidal action. As previously noted [20], connectedness can be considered similar to MiL in its reference to one's attachment to a work, to a role, or to shared projects and interests that keep one invested in living. Thus, their negative predictions for the role of SI could also be conceptually linked.

Taken together, these findings show that exploring the presence of MiL and the search for MiL contribute to refining the SB risk assessment. By widening the boundaries of diagnostic interviews to these two constructs, new entry points to SI could possibly be determined in both clinical and non-clinical populations [55], but particularly in populations that (1) can have silent/occult SI and (2) can abruptly experience out-of-the-ordinary experiences (e.g., veterans) [22].

Moreover, the presence of MiL and the search for MiL could constitute a useful target for psychotherapeutic interventions designed to decrease SB risk. These two constructs can be dealt with from different perspectives. Therapeutic modalities were initially systematized according to the classical assumptions of the existential–humanistic Logotherapy of Viktor E. Frankl [75]. Subsequently, Meaning-Centered Counseling, consisting of a cognitive-behavioral reformulation of Logotherapy [76], and Meaning-Centered Counseling and Therapy, consisting of an eclectic model that integrates different theories with MiL as its central and unifying theme [77], were proposed. Finally, a program aimed at achieving meaningful personal goals has been described [21], which, in patients with a borderline personality disorder, could be articulated with Dialectical Behavioral Therapy [20,49]. Although not specifically, the first three models [75–77] address both constructs, while the last model [20,21,49] is more focused on the presence of the Mil construct. Considering all these previous, precious, contributions (and after we have acquired more knowledge on the dynamic interplay of the two constructs), a specific approach for both the presence of Mil and the search for MiL could provide a promising psychotherapeutic area of study.

5. Limitations

This review has several limitations. First, it is based on studies of various natures. In qualitative and retrospective studies, clinical variables are not always readily available. Second, the studies investigated very heterogeneous populations. Some were conducted using non-clinical individuals of various ages and socio-professional conditions, while others used clinical populations with various psychiatric diagnoses, who were either outpatients or inpatients. Some studies also considered mixed samples of patients belonging to different age groups with various psychiatric diagnoses and in various stages of a given disorder. Third, these studies used varied instruments to examine the possible links between SB and the constructs in question. Furthermore, the SB risk was sometimes evaluated using differing methods. Given these factors, the data were often difficult to make generalizable.

We did not carry out a meta-analysis because the data from most of these studies did not permit such an approach. The studies used different measures and had differing outcomes, assessed patients at differing time points, and had several methodological problems, which often made the results difficult to interpret. Moreover, most of the studies considered nonhomogeneous samples, analyzed only a few variables, and did not include a control group. Finally, there are a limited number of articles in the literature concerning the topic of this review, particularly when distinguishing between the presence of MiL and the search for MiL.

6. Conclusions

In conclusion, considering the important limitations stated, MiL nonetheless emerges as a protective factor against suicidality. This has been demonstrated particularly for the MiL construct presence of MiL on SI and its inclusion among non-clinical psychiatric populations. These findings have clinical repercussions on SB prevention in both SB assessment and psychotherapeutic interventions. However, further research is needed to confirm the role of the presence of MiL and to clarify its interplay with the search for MiL, particularly in (1) clinical psychiatric populations (to possibly quantify their impacts on SB risk despite clinical conditions), (2) longitudinally designed cohorts, and (3) studies addressing SAs.

Author Contributions: A.C. drafted the primary manuscript, contributed to the conceptualization of the study, and participated to study selection/data collection; M.P. (Massimo Prelati) corrected/reviewed the manuscript, contributed to the conceptualization of the study, and participated to study selection/data collection; M.P. (Maurizio Pompili) corrected/reviewed the manuscript, conceptualized the study, supervised the work, and provided the intellectual impetus. All authors approved the final manuscript.

Funding: This research received no external funding.

Acknowledgments: The authors are grateful to A. Canuto, M. Baertschi, and K. Weber.

Conflicts of Interest: The authors declare no conflicts of interest.

References

1. Wang, M.C.; Richard Lightsey, O.; Pietruszka, T.; Uruk, A.C.; Wells, A.G. Purpose in life and reasons for living as mediators of the relationship between stress, coping, and suicidal behavior. *J. Posit. Psychol.* **2007**, *2*, 195–204. [CrossRef]
2. Frankl, V.E. *Man's Search for Meaning. From Death Camp to Existentialism*, 1st ed.; Beacon Press: New York, NY, USA, 1959.
3. Reker, G.T. Theoretical perspective, dimensions, and measurement of existential meaning. In *Exploring Existential Meaning: Optimizing Human Development Across the Life Span*; Recker, G.T., Chamberlain, K., Eds.; SAGE Publications Inc.: New York, NY, USA, 2000; pp. 39–55.
4. Park, C.L. Making sense of the meaning literature: An integrative review of meaning making and its effects on adjustment to stressful life events. *Psychol. Bull.* **2010**, *136*, 257–301. [CrossRef] [PubMed]
5. Wong, P.T.P. Introduction: A roadmap for meaning research and applications. In *The Human Quest for Meaning: Theories, Research, and Applications*; Wong, P., Ed.; Routledge, Taylor Francis Group: New York, NY, USA, London, UK 2012; pp. xxvii–xliv.
6. Glaw, X.; Kable, A.; Hazelton, M.; Inder, K. Meaning in life and meaning of life in mental health care: An integrative literature review. *Issues Ment. Health Nurs.* **2017**, *38*, 243–252. [CrossRef] [PubMed]
7. Martela, F.; Steger, M.F. The three meanings of meaning in life: Distinguishing coherence, purpose, and significance. *J. Posit. Psychol.* **2016**, *11*, 531–545. [CrossRef]
8. Steger, M.F. Experiencing meaning in life: Optimal functioning at the nexus of well-being, psychopathology, and spirituality. In *The Human Quest for Meaning: Theories, Research, and Applications*; Wong, P.T.P., Ed.; Routledge, Taylor Francis Group: New York, NY, USA; London, UK, 2012; pp. 165–184.

9. Steger, M. Meaning in life. In *The Oxford Handbook of Positive Psychology*; Lopez, S., Snyder, C., Eds.; Oxford University Press: Oxford, UK, 2009; pp. 679–688.
10. Steger, M.F.; Oishi, S.; Kesebir, S. Is a life without meaning satisfying? The moderating role of the search for meaning in satisfaction with life judgments. *J. Posit. Psychol.* **2011**, *6*, 173–180. [CrossRef]
11. Steger, M.; Kashdan, T. Search for meaning in life. In *Encyclopedia of Social Psychology*; Baumeister, R., Vohs, K., Eds.; Sage Publications: Thousand Oaks, CA, USA, 2007; pp. 783–785.
12. Frankl, V.E.; Crumbaugh, J.C.; Gerz, H.O.; Maholick, L.T. *Psychotherapy and Existentialism: Selected Papers on Logotherapy*; Simon and Schuster: New York, NY, USA, 1967; pp. 71–75.
13. Maddi, S.R. The search for meaning. In *Nebraska Symposium on Motivation*; Page, M., Ed.; University of Nebraska Press: Lincoln, NE, USA, 1970; pp. 137–186.
14. Baumeister, R.F. *Meanings of Life*; Guilford Press: New York, NY, USA, 1991.
15. Klinger, E. The search for meaning in evolutionary perspective and its clinical implications. In *The Human Quest for Meaning: A Handbook of Psychological Research and Clinical Application*; Wong, P.T.P., Fry, P.S., Eds.; Lawrence Erlbaum Associates: Mahwah, NJ, USA, 1998; pp. 25–70.
16. Steger, M.F.; Kashdan, T.B.; Sullivan, B.A.; Lorentz, D. Understanding the search for meaning in life: Personality, cognitive style, and the dynamic between seeking and experiencing meaning. *J. Pers.* **2008**, *76*, 199–228. [CrossRef]
17. Dezutter, J.; Casalin, S.; Wachholtz, A.; Luyckx, K.; Hekking, J.; Vandewiele, W. Meaning in life: An important factor for the psychological well-being of chronically ill patients? *Rehabil. Psychol.* **2013**, *58*, 334–341. [CrossRef]
18. Dezutter, J.; Luyckx, K.; Wachholtz, A. Meaning in life in chronic pain patients over time: Associations with pain experience and psychological well-being. *J. Behav. Med.* **2015**, *38*, 384–396. [CrossRef]
19. Marco, J.H.; Pérez, S.; García-Alandete, J. Meaning in life buffers the association between risk factors for suicide and hopelessness in participants with mental disorders. *J. Clin. Psychol.* **2016**, *72*, 689–700. [CrossRef]
20. Marco, J.H.; Pérez, S.; García-Alandete, J.; Moliner, R. Meaning in life in people with borderline personality disorder. *Clin. Psychol. Psychother.* **2017**, *24*, 162–170. [CrossRef]
21. Lapierre, S.; Dubé, M.; Bouffard, L.; Alain, M. Addressing suicidal ideations through the realization of meaningful personal goals. *Crisis* **2007**, *28*, 16–25. [CrossRef] [PubMed]
22. Denneson, L.M.; Teo, A.R.; Ganzini, L.; Helmer, D.A.; Bair, M.J.; Dobscha, S.K. Military veterans' experiences with suicidal ideation: Implications for intervention and prevention. *Suicide Life Threat. Behav.* **2015**, *45*, 399–414. [CrossRef] [PubMed]
23. Moher, D.; Liberati, A.; Tetzlaff, J.; Altman, D.G. Preferred Reporting Items for Systematic Reviews and Meta-Analyses: The PRISMA statement. *BMJ* **2009**, *339*, b2535. [CrossRef] [PubMed]
24. Higgins, J.P.T.; Green, S. *Cochrane Handbook for Systematic Reviews of Interventions Version 5.1.0 [Updated March 2011]*; The Cochrane Collaboration: London, UK, 2014.
25. Serafini, G.; Muzio, C.; Piccinini, G.; Flouri, E.; Ferrigno, G.; Pompili, M.; Girardi, P.; Amore, M. Life adversities and suicidal behavior in young individuals: A systematic review. *Eur. Child Adolesc. Psychiatry* **2015**, *24*, 1423–1446. [CrossRef] [PubMed]
26. Serafini, G.; Calcagno, P.; Lester, D.; Girardi, P.; Amore, M.; Pompili, M. Suicide risk in Alzheimer's disease: A systematic review. *Curr. Alzheimer Res.* **2016**, *13*, 1083–1099. [CrossRef]
27. Edwards, M.J.; Holden, R.R. Coping, meaning in life, and suicidal manifestations: Examining gender differences. *J. Clin. Psychol.* **2001**, *57*, 1517–1534. [CrossRef] [PubMed]
28. Orbach, I.; Mikulincer, M.; Gilboa-Schechtman, E.; Sirota, P. Mental pain and its relationship to suicidality and life meaning. *Suicide Life Threat. Behav.* **2003**, *33*, 231–241. [CrossRef]
29. Heisel, M.J.; Flett, G.L. Psychological resilience to suicide ideation among older adults. *Clin. Gerontol.* **2008**, *31*, 51–70. [CrossRef]
30. Bjerkeset, O.; Nordahl, H.M.; Romundstad, P.R.; Gunnell, D. PW01-253-personality traits, self-esteem and sense of meaning in life as predictors for suicide: The Norwegian HUNT cohort. *Eur. Psychiatry* **2010**, *25*, 1681. [CrossRef]
31. Kleiman, E.M.; Adams, L.M.; Kashdan, T.B.; Riskind, J.H. Gratitude and grit indirectly reduce risk of suicidal ideations by enhancing meaning in life: Evidence for a mediated moderation model. *J. Res. Personal.* **2013**, *47*, 539–546. [CrossRef]

32. Henry, K.L.; Lovegrove, P.J.; Steger, M.F.; Chen, P.Y.; Cigularov, K.P.; Tomazic, R.G. The potential role of meaning in life in the relationship between bullying victimization and suicidal ideation. *J. Youth Adolesc.* **2014**, *43*, 221–232. [CrossRef] [PubMed]
33. Wilchek-Aviad, Y. Meaning in life and suicidal tendency among immigrant (Ethiopian) youth and native-born Israeli youth. *J. Immigr. Minor. Health* **2015**, *17*, 1041–1048. [CrossRef] [PubMed]
34. Heisel, M.J.; Flett, G.L. Does recognition of meaning in life confer resiliency to suicide ideation among community-residing older adults? A longitudinal investigation. *Am. J. Geriatr. Psychiatry* **2016**, *24*, 455–466. [CrossRef] [PubMed]
35. Heisel, M.J.; Neufeld, E.; Flett, G.L. Reasons for living, meaning in life, and suicide ideation: Investigating the roles of key positive psychological factors in reducing suicide risk in community-residing older adults. *Aging Ment. Health* **2016**, *20*, 195–207. [CrossRef] [PubMed]
36. Wilchek-Aviad, Y.; Malka, M. Religiosity, meaning in life and suicidal tendency among Jews. *J. Relig. Health* **2016**, *55*, 480–494. [CrossRef] [PubMed]
37. Wilchek-Aviad, Y.; Ne'eman-Haviv, V.; Malka, M. Connection between suicidal ideation, life meaning, and leisure time activities. *Deviant Behav.* **2017**, *38*, 621–632. [CrossRef]
38. Wilchek-Aviad, Y.; Ne'eman-Haviv, V. The relation between a sense of meaning in life and suicide potential among disadvantaged adolescent girls. *Int. J. Offender Ther. Comp. Criminol.* **2018**, *62*, 1474–1487. [CrossRef] [PubMed]
39. Schnell, T.; Gerstner, R.; Krampe, H. Crisis of meaning predicts suicidality in youth independently of depression. *Crisis* **2018**, *39*, 294–303. [CrossRef] [PubMed]
40. Liu, Y.; Usman, M.; Zhang, J.; Gul, H. Making sense of Chinese employees' suicidal ideation: A psychological strain—Life Meaning Model. *Psychol. Rep.* **2018**. [CrossRef]
41. Testoni, I.; Russotto, S.; Zamperini, A.; De Leo, D. Addiction and religiosity in facing suicide: A qualitative study on meaning of life and death among homeless people. *Ment. Illn.* **2018**, *10*, 16–24. [CrossRef] [PubMed]
42. Moore, S.L. A phenomenological study of meaning in life in suicidal older adults. *Arch. Psychiatr. Nurs.* **1997**, *11*, 29–36. [CrossRef]
43. Heisel, M.J.; Flett, G.L. Purpose in life, satisfaction with life, and suicide ideation in a clinical sample. *J. Psychopathol. Behav. Assess.* **2004**, *26*, 127–135. [CrossRef]
44. Van Orden, K.A.; Bamonti, P.M.; King, D.A.; Duberstein, P.R. Does perceived burdensomeness erode meaning in life among older adults? *Aging Ment. Health* **2012**, *16*, 855–860. [CrossRef] [PubMed]
45. Holm, A.L.; Lyberg, A.; Berggren, I.; Åström, S.; Severinsson, E. Going around in a circle: A Norwegian study of suicidal experiences in old age. *Nurs. Res. Pract.* **2014**, *2014*, 734635. [CrossRef] [PubMed]
46. García-Alandete, J.; Salvador, M.; José, H.; Pérez Rodríguez, S. Predicting role of the meaning in life on depression, hopelessness, and suicide risk among borderline personality disorder patients. *Univ. Psychol.* **2014**, *13*, 1545–1555. [CrossRef]
47. Van Orden, K.A.; Wiktorsson, S.; Duberstein, P.; Berg, A.I.; Fässberg, M.M.; Waern, M. Reasons for attempted suicide in later life. *Am. J. Geriatr. Psychiatry* **2015**, *23*, 536–544. [CrossRef]
48. Braden, A.; Overholser, J.; Fisher, L.; Ridley, J. Life meaning is associated with suicidal ideation among depressed veterans. *Death Stud.* **2015**, *39*, 24–29. [CrossRef]
49. Marco, J.H.; Guillén, V.; Botella, C. The buffer role of meaning in life in hopelessness in women with borderline personality disorders. *Psychiatry Res.* **2017**, *247*, 120–124. [CrossRef]
50. Marco, J.H.; Cañabate, M.; Pérez, S.; Llorca, G. Associations among meaning in life, body image, psychopathology, and suicide ideation in Spanish participants with eating disorders. *J. Clin. Psychol.* **2017**, *73*, 1768–1781. [CrossRef]
51. Perez Rodriguez, S.; Marco Salvador, J.H.; García-Alandete, J. The role of hopelessness and meaning in life in a clinical sample with non-suicidal self-injury and suicide attempts. *Psicothema* **2017**, *29*, 323–328.
52. Pérez, S.; Marco, J.H.; García-Alandete, J. Psychopathological differences between suicide ideators and suicide attempters in patients with mental disorders. *Clin. Psychol. Psychother.* **2017**, *24*, 1002–1013. [CrossRef]
53. Lamis, D.A.; Kapoor, S.; Evans, A.P. Childhood sexual abuse and suicidal ideation among bipolar patients: Existential but not religious well-being as a protective factor. *Suicide Life Threat. Behav.* **2018**, *49*, 401–412. [CrossRef]
54. Florez, I.A.; Allbaugh, L.J.; Harris, C.E.; Schwartz, A.C.; Kaslow, N.J. Suicidal ideation and hopelessness in PTSD: Spiritual well-being mediates outcomes over time. *Anxiety Stress Coping* **2018**, *31*, 46–58. [CrossRef]

55. Kleiman, E.M.; Beaver, J.K. A meaningful life is worth living: Meaning in life as a suicide resiliency factor. *Psychiatry Res.* **2013**, *210*, 934–939. [CrossRef]
56. Kim, H.M.; Levine, D.S.; Pfeiffer, P.N.; Blow, A.J.; Marchiondo, C.; Walters, H.; Valenstein, M. Postdeployment suicide risk increases over a 6-month period: Predictors of increased risk among Midwestern Army National Guard soldiers. *Suicide Life Threat. Behav.* **2017**, *47*, 421–435. [CrossRef]
57. Collins, K.R.; Legendre, M.N.; Stritzke, W.G.; Page, A.C. Experimentally-enhanced perceptions of meaning confer resilience to the interpersonal adversity implicated in suicide risk. *J. Behav. Ther. Exp. Psychiatry* **2018**, *61*, 142–149. [CrossRef]
58. Sinclair, S.; Bryan, C.J.; Bryan, A.O. Meaning in life as a protective factor for the emergence of suicide ideation that leads to suicide attempts among military personnel and veterans with elevated PTSD and depression. *Int. J. Cogn. Ther.* **2016**, *9*, 87–98. [CrossRef]
59. Lu, H.F.; Sheng, W.H.; Liao, S.C.; Chang, N.T.; Wu, P.Y.; Yang, Y.L.; Hsiao, F.H. The changes and the predictors of suicide ideation and suicide attempt among HIV-positive patients at 6–12 months post diagnosis: A longitudinal study. *J. Adv. Nurs.* **2018**, *75*, 573–584. [CrossRef]
60. Crumbaugh, J.C.; Maholick, L.T. *Manual of Instructions for the Purpose-in-Life Test*; Viktor Frankl Institute of Logotherapy: Saratoga, CA, USA, 1969.
61. García-Alandete, J.; Martínez, E.R.; Nohales, P.S. Estructura Factorial y Consistencia Interna de una Versión Española del Purpose-In-Life Test [Factorial Structure and Internal Consistency of a Spanish Version of the Purpose in Life Test]. *Univ. Psychol.* **2013**, *12*, 517–530. [CrossRef]
62. Heisel, M.J.; Flett, G.L. The development and initial validation of the Geriatric Suicide Ideation Scale. *Am. J. Geriatr. Psychiatry* **2006**, *14*, 742–751. [CrossRef]
63. Heisel, M.J. Assessing experienced meaning in life among older adults: The development and initial validation of the EMIL. *Int. Psychogeriatr.* **2009**, *21*, S172–S173.
64. Batista, J.; Almond, R. The development of meaning in life. *Psychiatry* **1973**, *36*, 409–427. [CrossRef]
65. Debats, D.L. Measurement of Personal Meaning: The Psychometric Properties of the Life Regard Index. In *The Human Quest for Meaning: A Handbook of Psychological Research and Clinical Applications*; Wong, P.T.P., Fry, P.S., Eds.; Lawrence Erlbaum Associates Publishers: Mahwah, NJ, USA, 1998; pp. 237–259.
66. Antonovsky, A. The structure and properties of the sense of coherence scale. *Soc. Sci. Med.* **1993**, *36*, 725–733. [CrossRef]
67. Schnell, T. The Sources of Meaning and Meaning in Life Questionnaire (SoMe): Relations to demographics and well-being. *J. Posit. Psychol.* **2009**, *4*, 483–499. [CrossRef]
68. Morgan, J.; Farsides, T. Measuring meaning in life. *J. Happiness Stud.* **2009**, *10*, 197–214. [CrossRef]
69. Ellison, C.W. Spiritual well-being: Conceptualization and measurement. *J. Psychol. Theol.* **1983**, *11*, 330–338. [CrossRef]
70. Steger, M.F.; Frazier, P.; Oishi, S.; Kaler, M. The meaning in life questionnaire: Assessing the presence of and search for meaning in life. *J. Couns. Psychol.* **2006**, *53*, 80–93. [CrossRef]
71. Joiner, T.E. *Why People Die by Suicide*; Harvard University Press: Cambridge, MA, USA, 2005.
72. Van Orden, K.A.; Witte, T.K.; Cukrowicz, K.C.; Braithwaite, S.R.; Selby, E.A.; Joiner, T.E., Jr. The interpersonal theory of suicide. *Psychol. Rev.* **2010**, *117*, 575–600. [CrossRef]
73. Osman, A.; Bagge, C.L.; Gutierrez, P.M.; Konick, L.C.; Kopper, B.A.; Barrios, F.X. The Suicidal Behaviors Questionnaire-Revised (SBQ-R): Validation with clinical and nonclinical samples. *Assessment* **2001**, *8*, 443–454. [CrossRef]
74. Klonsky, D.E.; May, A.M. The Three-Step Theory (3ST): A New Theory of Suicide Rooted in the "Ideation-to-Action" Framework. *Int. J. Cogn. Ther.* **2015**, *8*, 114–129. [CrossRef]
75. Frankl, V.E. *The Will to Meaning: Foundations and Applications of Logotherapy*; New American Library: New York, NY, USA, 1988.
76. Wong, P.T.P. Meaning-centered counseling: A cognitive-behavioral approach to Logotherapy. *Int. Forum Logother.* **1997**, *20*, 85–94.
77. Wong, P.T.P. Towards an integrative model of meaning-centered counseling and therapy. *Int. Forum Logother.* **1998**, *22*, 47–55.

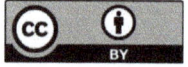

© 2019 by the authors. Licensee MDPI, Basel, Switzerland. This article is an open access article distributed under the terms and conditions of the Creative Commons Attribution (CC BY) license (http://creativecommons.org/licenses/by/4.0/).

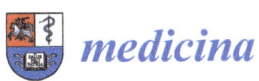

Review

Can Anhedonia Be Considered a Suicide Risk Factor? A Review of the Literature

Luca Bonanni [1], Flavia Gualtieri [1], David Lester [2], Giulia Falcone [1], Adele Nardella [1], Andrea Fiorillo [3] and Maurizio Pompili [4,*]

1. Psychiatry Residency Training Program, Faculty of Medicine and Psychology, Sapienza University of Rome, 00189 Rome, Italy
2. Psychology Program, Stockton University, Galloway, NJ 08205, USA
3. Department of Psychiatry, University of Campania Luigi Vanvitelli, 80138 Naples, Italy
4. Department of Neurosciences, Mental Health and Sensory Organs, Suicide Prevention Center, Sant'Andrea Hospital, Sapienza University of Rome, 00189 Rome, Italy
* Correspondence: maurizio.pompili@uniroma1.it; Tel.: +39-06-3377-5675; Fax: +39-06-3377-5342

Received: 11 June 2019; Accepted: 6 August 2019; Published: 9 August 2019

Abstract: *Background and Objectives*: At present, data collected from the literature about suicide and anhedonia are controversial. Some studies have shown that low levels of anhedonia are associated with serious suicide attempts and death by suicide, while other studies have shown that high levels of anhedonia are associated with suicide. *Materials and Methods*: For this review, we searched PubMed, Medline, and ScienceDirect for clinical studies published from 1 January 1990 to 31 December 2018 with the following search terms used in the title or in the abstract: "anhedonia AND suicid*." We obtained a total of 155 articles; 133 items were excluded using specific exclusion criteria, the remaining 22 articles included were divided into six groups based on the psychiatric diagnosis: mood disorders, schizophrenia spectrum disorders, post-traumatic stress disorder (PTSD), other diagnoses, attempted suicides, and others (healthy subjects). *Results*: The results of this review reveal inconsistencies. Some studies reported that high anhedonia scores were associated with suicidal behavior (regardless of the diagnosis), while other studies found that low anhedonia scores were associated with suicidal behavior, and a few studies reported no association. The most consistent association between anhedonia and suicidal behavior was found for affective disorders (7 of 7 studies reported a significant positive association) and for PTSD (3 of 3 studies reported a positive association). In the two studies of patients with schizophrenia, one found no association, and one found a negative association. For patients who attempted suicide (undiagnosed), one study found a positive association, one a positive association only for depressed attempters, and one a negative association. *Conclusions*: We found the most consistent positive association for patients with affective disorders and PTSD, indicating that the assessment of anhedonia may be useful in the evaluation of suicidal risk.

Keywords: anhedonia; PTSD; suicide; suicide risk; suicidal behavior

---

1. Introduction

Suicide is a severe public health problem with more than one million deaths reported each year worldwide [1] and with nearly 20 times more people attempting suicide each year [2]. Moreover, suicide ranks among the ten major causes of death worldwide and is a leading cause of death among youth and young adults in many countries [3–6]. Given the prevalence of suicidal ideation and behaviors and the associated medical expenses, it is important to know what factors lead to both suicidal thoughts and suicide attempts in order to identify reliably those transitioning from suicidal ideation to fatal suicidal behaviors [7]. Developing this ability will inform suicide risk assessment methods and early intervention tools.

The MATRICS consensus conference on negative symptoms, convened under the auspices of the National Institutes of Mental Health (NIMH) in 2005, suggested that there are five general categories of negative symptoms: avolition, anhedonia, asociality, affective blunting, and alogia. The most common negative symptoms are avolition and anhedonia, and one of the most persistent negative symptoms is anhedonia, that is not experiencing pleasure or having the ability to obtain pleasure from activities or interpersonal relationships. In DSM-5, anhedonia is defined as "Lack of enjoyment from, engagement in, or energy for life's experiences; deficits in the capacity to feel pleasure and take an interest in things." Anhedonia is present in both patients with schizophrenia and patients with depression. It is estimated that half of schizophrenia patients experience anhedonia, although estimates of its prevalence vary greatly. Anhedonia and social isolation predict schizophrenia in high-risk populations [8].

Lately, there has been a growing interest in anhedonia with the evidence suggesting that this symptom may be a unique predictor of psychopathology [9], including suicidality [10–12]. For example, a study of 40 patients with depression and 20 controls showed that individuals who had suicidal ideation and previous suicidal attempts were less likely to respond to rewarding stimuli on a task designed to assess the presence of anhedonia [12].

The results of the research, however, are inconsistent. Some research has shown that low levels of anhedonia are associated with serious suicide attempts and death by suicide [13,14], while other research has shown that high levels of anhedonia are associated with suicide [15–18]. A study conducted by Winer et al. [19] showed that anhedonia is associated with suicidal ideation but not with previous suicide attempts. Regarding the observed relationship between anhedonia and suicidal behavior, Nock and Kazdin [10] suggested that anhedonia is experienced as an intolerable state leading to suicidal behavior to escape a current stressor. Other research shows that those who think of suicide feel less pleasure and are focused on efforts to avoid psychological pain [12], and a reduction in psychological pain has been observed when individuals engage in suicidal behavior [20]. Some studies have suggested that anhedonia is a modifiable clinical factor associated with suicidal ideation, independently of depressive symptoms [21].

As mentioned above, several studies have shown that anhedonia is related to an increased risk of suicide, while others have claimed the opposite. This discrepancy can be understood using the following considerations [22]. First, anhedonia can be considered either as a trait or as a state. When anhedonia is a state, presenting and persisting as a symptom of a specific psychiatric disorder and, particularly, depression, it may be a risk factor for suicide. When it is considered as a trait, with long-term stability and not associated with depression, it may not act as a risk factor for suicide or it may be associated with a low risk of suicide [23]. Also significant is the difference between consummatory and anticipatory anhedonia [24], although this is rarely taken into consideration. A deficit in consummatory pleasure can characterize endogenomorphic depression, a subtype of depression associated with a higher risk of suicide [25]. Moreover, there is not just one but several types of suicide risk: suicidal ideation, suicide attempt (recent or not), and completed suicide. In addition, there is a great deal of difference in the methodology used in studies proposing to demonstrate a correlation between anhedonia and suicide risk which should be kept in mind. In fact, these studies do not have homogeneity in the types of sample chosen (differentiating for example by age, gender, etc.,) as well as a control of the confounding variables (such as outpatients or inpatients) and a control for depression level (that is, the effect of the anhedonia independently of depression) [22].

Although some medications, such as lithium [26,27] and clozapine [27,28], as well as psychotherapy, have shown effectiveness in managing suicidal behavior, the rates of suicidal ideation, suicide attempts, and completed suicides have not substantially decreased in recent years [29]. Hence, it will be useful to know in more detail the risk factors for suicide, such as anhedonia, in order to create alternative suicide prevention tactics, and the present review of the literature tries to understand the association between suicidal behaviors and anhedonia.

2. Materials and Methods

For this review, we searched PubMed, Medline, and ScienceDirect for clinical studies published from 1 January 1990 to 31 December 2018 with the following search terms used in the title or in the abstract: "anhedonia AND suicid*". Initially, two reviewers screened the abstracts of studies identified for eligibility with 100% agreement, and then another reviewer assessed the included studies. All three reviewers discussed any disagreements identified and reached an agreement before proceeding. We obtained a total of 155 articles of which 133 articles were excluded using the following exclusion criteria: reviews or meta-analyses (21), case reports (2), letters/opinions (1), non-psychiatric studies (6) or unfocused (98), and studies conducted on adolescents (5). The 22 articles included in this review were divided into six groups based on the psychiatric diagnosis: mood disorders, schizophrenia spectrum disorders, post-traumatic stress disorder, other diagnoses (such as anxiety disorders), attempted suicide, and others (that is, without a psychiatric diagnosis). Details of the trials included (study design, sample size, criteria, objectives, evaluation tools, outcomes) were extracted and are reported in Table 1.

Table 1. Summary of reports on suicide behavior and anhedonia.

Reference	Study Design	Sample	Criteria	Mood Disorder Objectives	Methods	Results
Zielinski et al. 2017	Prospective longitudinal study	187 participants	Participants (mean age = 34.41) with a history of non-suicidal self-injury or previous suicide attempts	To verify if modifications in depressive symptoms and anhedonia can be considered as predictive factors of suicide and self-harm behavior	- DASS-21 © to assess depressive symptoms - SLIPS ¥ to evaluate anhedonia - SBQ-R ⊥ to assess several dimensions of suicidal risk - OSI£ to evaluate self-harm behavior	Anhedonia scores were higher in those with prior suicide attempts than in those with a history of non-suicidal self-injury. Depressive symptoms predicted suicidal behavior directly and also via mediation through anhedonia
Ballard et al. 2017	Retrospective longitudinal study	100 participants	Patients (18–65 years) affected by treatment-resistant major depressive disorder (n = 65) or bipolar disorder without psychotic features (n = 35) recruited from several clinical trials of ketamine	To evaluate the relationship between the decrease of suicidal ideation after ketamine administration and the reduction of anhedonia	- BDI *-II and the SHAPS # to assess anhedonia - SSI5 ⊘ to assess suicidal ideation	At baseline, anhedonia scores were associated with suicidal ideation. After administration of ketamine, both suicidal ideation and anhedonia declined. The change in anhedonia accounted for an additional 13% of the variance for changes in suicidal thoughts beyond the effects of depressive symptoms
Ballard et al. 2016	Prospective study from the STEP-BD study (4360 patients)	530 participants	Subjects who attempted or died by suicide (n = 103) vs. controls (n = 427)	To individualize which clinical dimensions (suicidal ideation, loss of interest, anxiety, psychomotor agitation, high-risk behavior) increase before suicidal conduct	- Clinical Monitoring Form (CMF) for clinic evaluation	Patients with suicidal behavior had an elevation of all symptoms, including loss of interest. Suicidal ideation and loss of interest were highly intense in the months before the suicidal behavior and can be considered a risk factor for suicidal behavior in bipolar patients
Xie et al. 2014	Cross-sectional study	60 participants	Participants (18–60 years) included patients affected by major depressive disorder (n = 40) vs. control subjects without psychiatric disorder (n = 20). Based on BSS scores, psychiatric patients were divided into two subgroups: high suicidal ideation (HSI) group and low suicidal ideation (LSI) group	To analyze the association between anhedonia, pain avoidance motivation, and suicidal ideation	- BDI *-II to assess depressive symptoms - BSS$ for suicidal ideation - PAS ¢ and TDPPS € to evaluate physical and mental pain - MID · and AID §	In AID task, the HSI had longer response times (RTs) under the reward condition than those under the punishment condition ($p = 0.002$); the LSI group and control groups had shorter RTs under the reward condition than those under the neutral condition ($p < 0.001$ and $p = 0.008$, respectively); the LSI group had shorter RTs under the reward condition than under the punishment condition ($p = 0.003$). Pain arousal ($p < 0.01$) and BSS scores were significantly negatively correlated with differences in RTs between neutral and reward conditions and positively correlated with differences in RTs between neutral and punishment conditions. The AID was the best task for detection of hedonic approach to experiences and of pain avoidance so that a reduced motivation to experience anhedonia and an increased one to avoid pain can be considered reliable predictors of suicidal behavior
Spijker et al. 2010	Prospective epidemiologic survey	586 participants	Data were extracted from the Netherlands Mental Health Survey and Incidence Study (NEMESIS). Participants were adults (18–64 years) with a depressive spectrum disorder (≥2 depressive symptoms—according to Composite International Diagnostic Interview—CIDI)	To individuate determinants of suicidality (suicidal ideation and suicide attempts) and compare these two factors	- One item of the CIDI to evaluate suicidal ideation and suicide attempts	Suicidal ideation was influenced by different clinical features: longer duration of depression—13 months—($p = 0.01$), anhedonia ($p = 0.05$), feeling worthless ($p = 0.03$), comorbid anxiety ($p < 0.01$), previous suicidal ideation ($p < 0.001$), and use of professional care ($p = 0.05$). Anxiety, suicidal ideation, previous suicide attempts, and living alone were significantly related with suicide attempts (respectively $p = 0.01$; $p = 0.05$; $p < 0.01$; $p = 0.02$)

Table 1. Cont.

Reference	Study Design	Sample	Criteria	Objectives	Methods	Results
Oei et al. 1990	Cross-sectional study	46 participants	Patients (18–65 years) with depressive symptoms (according to DSM-III) were recruited from Department of Psychiatry of the University Hospital in Utrecht (The Netherlands)	To evaluate the relationship between anhedonia, suicidal behavior, and dexamethasone non suppression	- HDRS § and MADRS † for depression - BSS $ for suicidal ideation - CPAS ° to assess anhedonia - STAI ≠ for anxiety -Dexamethasone (DEX) Suppression	The combination of anhedonia ($p < 0.001$), suicidal ideation ($p < 0.05$), and DEX-non-suppression ($p < 0.05$) identified a subgroup of patients affected by depressive disorder who presented three positive symptoms
Fawcett et al. 1990	Prospective study	954 participants	954 subjects (mean age = 38.1) affected by major affective disorder (according to Research Diagnostic Criteria)		- Schedules for affective disorders and schizophrenia (SADS)	3% of the subjects committed suicide: 41% of the patients died during the first year of follow-up. Suicide was associated with anhedonia ($p = 0.05$) in the 12-month follow-up

Schizophrenic Spectrum Disorder

Reference	Study Design	Sample	Criteria	Objectives	Methods	Results
Jahn et al. 2016	Prospective study	162 participants	Patients (mean age = 46.84) affected by schizophrenia or schizoaffective disorder (according to DSM-IV)	To examine the role of social functioning on suicidal ideation	- BPRS †† (24-item expanded version) to assess symptoms - RPS Σ and Social Closeness Scale from MPQ - SC ° for social role functioning - CAINS ± to assess negative symptoms	Motivation and pleasure-related negative symptoms influenced the relationship between social role functioning and suicidal ideation ($p < 0.001$). A low level of suicidal ideation was associated with better social role functioning in patients who had low motivation and pleasure-related negative symptoms
Loas et al. 2009	Prospective study	150 participants	150 in- or outpatients affected by chronic schizophrenia were included from April 1991 to July 1995 and followed-up for 14 years	To compare clinical symptoms (positive and negative) of schizophrenic patients who died by suicide vs. patients who died by other causes	- BPRS †† - CPAS ° to assess anhedonia - BDI *·II - PANSS ◊	Patients who died from suicide had a shorter duration of illness, and a higher level of education vs. patients died from other causes ($p = 0.02$). Negative symptoms and deficit syndrome can be considered as protective factors in schizophrenia.Anhedonia was associated with a higher risk of suicide in schizophrenia ($p = 0.19$)

Post-Traumatic Stress Disorder

Reference	Study Design	Sample	Criteria	Objectives	Methods	Results
Spitzer et al. 2018	Cross-sectional study	373 participants	Psychology undergraduates students (mean age = 19.9) enrolled in a public university in the southeastern United States who satisfied criterion A of PTSD (DSM-5)	To analyze the association between PTSD dimensionality (based on the six-factor anhedonia model) and acquired capability for suicide (including fearlessness of pain involved in dying and fearlessness about death)	- FOP ** and FAD ∞ - DSM-5 to assess the diagnosis of PTSD - BDI *·II	Anhedonia cluster symptoms of PTSD was significantly related to the fearlessness of pain involved in dying ($p = 0.04$) and also fearlessness about death ($p = 0.03$)
Guina et al. 2017	Cross-sectional self-report survey	480 participants	Adults outpatients recruited at a military medical center with previous trauma	To investigate the relationships between suicide attempts and PTSD, trauma types, demographics, use of substance and benzodiazepine prescriptions	- Diagnostic and Statistical Manual of Mental Disorders -5(DSM-5) to assess the diagnosis of PTSD and to evaluate suicide attempts, previous traumatic events and abuse of alcohol or drugs	Suicide attempts were significantly associated with severity of PTSD symptom ($p < 0.0001$), childhood physical abuse ($p = 0.0002$), violent death of a loved one ($p = 0.0037$), childhood neglect ($p = 0.0099$), childhood sexual abuse ($p = 0.0246$), substance and alcohol problems (respectively $p = 0.0189$ and $p = 0.0128$), and benzodiazepine prescriptions ($p = 0.0006$)
Chen et al. 2017	Survey	36,309 participants	Participants (≥18 years) were recruited in 2012–2013. A sample of 23,936 subjects (2457 veterans) and 21,479 non-veterans) had a history of at least a traumatic event	To evaluate the clinical dimension of PTSD and its relationship with suicide attempts	- Lifetime suicide attempts-AUDADIS -5 ° to assess the diagnosis of PTSD	PTSD can be considered as a risk factor for suicide attempts and anhedonia. Anhedonia was recognized as a latent factor of PTSD and had a statistically significant effect on suicide attempts ($p < 0.05$)

Table 1. Cont.

Reference	Study Design	Sample	Criteria	Objectives	Methods	Results
				Other Diagnoses		
Hawes et al. 2018	Prospective study	395 participants	Participants (≥18 years) recruited from three adult psychiatric outpatient centers in New York City between January 2016 and March 2017	To explore the different effects of chronic vs. acute anhedonia on suicidal ideation and lifetime suicide attempts	- SHAPS [#] to assess anhedonia; - BDI *-II to assess depression; - STAI to assess anxiety; - $ BSS and [§] C-SSRS to assess severity of suicidal ideation and history of suicide attempts;	Recent changes in the capacity to experience pleasure is better for predicting near-term suicidal ideation than is chronic anhedonia. The acutely anhedonic group reported greater severity of suicidal ideation in the past-week ($p = 0.02$) and past-month ($p = 0.04$)
Loas et al. 2016	Cross-sectional study	122 participants	122 adult patients (mean age = 44.64) recruited between 2010 and 2013 in the Psychiatric Unit of the CHU of Amiens. Subjects had a diagnosis of mood disorder (n = 37) or anxiety disorder (n = 85) according to ICD-10. Forty-one patients were admitted for a suicide attempt	To explore the association between anhedonia, alexithymia, impulsivity, suicidal ideation, recent suicide attempt, C-Reactive Protein (CRP) and serum lipid profile	- TAS-20 [ॱ] for alexithymia - BIS-10 [†] for impulsivity - Subscales of the Temporal Experience Pleasure Scale for trait anhedonia - BDI *-II for anhedonia, depression and suicidal ideation - Blood samples for CRP and serum lipid profile (between 7:00 and 8:30 a.m. after at least 12 h of fast)	Anhedonia was related to low total cholesterol level ($p = 0.043$) and low triglycerides level ($p = 0.077$). There was an association between a low level of HDL cholesterol and high suicidal ideation ($p = 0.015$). Patients who committed suicide presented a higher level of CRP vs. patients without suicidal behavior ($p = 0.033$)
Winer et al. 2014	Prospective cohort study	1529 participants	Adult inpatients (mean age: 35.55 years) of a private, not-for-profit Psychiatric structure in the southern United States recruited between April 2008 and August 2011. Participants were affected by: depressive disorder (53.0%); bipolar disorder (16.06%); anxiety disorder (4.86%)	To investigate the association between suicidality and anhedonia	- BDI *-II (Anhedonia, depression symptoms and suicidal ideation were assessed at admission and discharge)	Anhedonia was associated with suicidality at baseline ($p = 0.001$) and at the end of hospitalization ($p = 0.001$). Change in anhedonia from baseline to termination predicted a change in suicidality
				Attempted Suicides		
Reference	Study Design	Sample	Criteria	Objectives	Methods	Results
Yaseen et al. 2016	Cross-sectional analysis	135 participants	Attempted suicides or high-risk patients admitted to an emergency room at Mount Sinai Beth Israel Hospital (New York)	To explore the association of anhedonia with suicidal ideation in attempted suicides and high-risk patients	- C-SSRS [§] to assess suicidal behavior - Items 4 and 12 of BDI *-II to assess anhedonia	Prior suicidal ideation was significantly associated with anhedonia, anxiety, and feelings of entrapment. Entrapment and anhedonia were independently associated also with the severity of suicidal ideation
Loas 2007	Follow-up study	106 participants	Attempted suicides admitted to the Hospital Nord d'Amiens	To predict suicide in a sample of attempted suicides	- PAS [%] to assess anhedonia	Patients who died from suicide in 6.5-year follow-up had lower anhedonia scores than those who did not die
Loas et al. 2000	Cross-sectional study	207 participants	Depressed patients (n = 73) and not-depressed patients (n = 30) admitted to the Centre Hospitalier Universitaire (CHU) Nord d'Amiens after a suicide attempt from September 1993 to August 1996 vs. 104 control subjects	To assess the effect of anhedonia on suicide and parasuicide in patients with depressive disorder and in healthy subjects	- CPAS [º] to assess anhedonia - BDI *-II to evaluate depression	Level of anhedonia was higher in depressed attempters vs. not-depressed attempters ($p < 0.001$) and vs. controls ($p < 0.001$). There was no difference in PAS score between healthy subjects and non-depressed attempters ($p < 0.05$)

Table 1. Cont.

Reference	Study Design	Sample	Criteria	Objectives	Methods	Results
						Others
Daghigh et al. 2018	Cross-sectional study	404 participants	Students of Kashan University (center of Persia)	To replicate in an Iranian sample finding of the association between anhedonia, suicide ideation and suicide attempts	- SLIPS ¥ for anhedonia - CES-D ¢ for depression - SBQ-R for suicidal behavior	Anhedonia was associated with suicidal risk ($p = 0.030$), independent of other symptoms of depression, and with suicide attempts ($p = 0.000$)
Loas et al. 2018	Cross-sectional study	557 participants	Participants were physicians	To explore the relationship between suicidality and anhedonia in a general population	- An abridged version of BDI *-13	Anhedonia was associated with both suicidal ideation ($p = 0.001$) and suicide attempts ($p = 0.001$). Anhedonia influenced the relationship between suicidal ideation and perceived burdensomeness ($p = 0.001$) and thwarted belongingness ($p = 0.001$). Suicide attempts were mediated only by thwarted belongingness. "Dissatisfaction" and "work inhibition" (two different component of anhedonia) can influence respectively suicidal ideation (lifetime-$p = 0.003$; recent- $p = 0.001$) and suicide attempts ($p = 0.001$)
Winer et al. 2016	Cross-sectional study	1122 participants	Undergraduate students (18–36 years) of a public university in the Southern United States	To assess the relationship between anhedonia, suicidal ideation, and suicide attempt	- SLIPS ¥ for anhedonia - CES-D ¢ for depression - SBQ-R ↓ for suicidal behavior	Suicidal ideation was influenced by anhedonia ($p < 0.05$). Anhedonia was not associated with suicide attempts ($p = 0.33$). Other depressive symptoms presented a correlation with suicide attempts ($p < 0.001$)
Loas et al. 1995	Cross-sectional study	224 participants	Healthy adult subjects of the Picardie (region of France) were included	To investigate the association between anhedonia, depression, and suicidal risk	- CPAS ° to assess anhedonia - BDI *-II to evaluate depression	There was no association between anhedonia and depression or anhedonia and suicidal ideation ($p = ns$)

§ AID: Affective Incentive Delay; * AUDADIS-5: The Alcohol Use Disorder and Associated Disabilities Interview Schedule; * BDI: Beck Depression Inventory; ¶ BIS-10: Barratt impulsivity scale; ↔ BPRS: Brief Psychiatric Rating Scale; $ BSS: Beck Scale for Suicide Ideation; ‡ CAINS: Clinical Assessment Interview for Negative Symptoms; ⁶ CES-D: Center of Epidemiological Studies Depression Scale; ³ C-SSRS: Columbia Suicide Severity Rating Scale; ° CPAS: Chapman Physical Anhedonia Scale; © DASS: Depression Anxiety Stress Scale; ∞ FAD: Fearlessness About Death; ↑ FDI-24: Future Disposition Inventory-24; ⁎ FOP: Scales for Fearlessness of Pain Involved in Dying; ⁸ HDRS: Hamilton Rating Scale for depression; † MADRS: Montgomery–Asberg Depression Rating Scale; ~ MID: Monetary Incentive Delay; ○ MPQ-SC: Multidimensional Personality Questionnaire; € OSI: Ottawa Self-Injury Inventory-Clinical; ○ PANSS: Positive and Negative Syndrome Scale; % PAS: Psychache Scale; Σ RFS: Role Functioning Scale; ↓ SBQ-R: Suicide Behaviors Questionnaire-Revised; # SHAPS: Snaith–Hamilton Pleasure Scale; ¥ SLIPS: Specific Loss of Interest and Pleasure Scale; ⊘ SSI5: Scale for Suicide Ideation; % STAI: State-Trait-Anxiety Inventory; ⁿ TAS-20: 20-item Toronto Alexithymia Scale; ᵠ TDPPS: Three-Dimensional Psychological Pain Scale.

3. Results

3.1. Affective Disorders

In a retrospective longitudinal study, Ballard et al. [21] studied 100 treatment-resistant patients with major depressive disorder ($n = 65$) or bipolar disorder ($n = 35$) using data from several clinical trials of ketamine to evaluate whether anhedonia can be considered a clinical correlate of suicidal thoughts. At baseline, anhedonia measured both by the Snaith–Hamilton Pleasure Scale (SHAPS) scale and the anhedonia subscale of the Beck Depression Inventory (BDI) was associated with suicidal ideation. A reduction in suicidal thoughts 230 min after the administration of ketamine was associated with a reduction in anhedonia, independently of a reduction in depressive symptoms. The change in anhedonia accounted for an additional 13% of the variance for changes in suicidal thoughts beyond the effects of depressive symptoms.

In a prospective longitudinal study of 187 adult patients with suicidal and/or non-suicidal self-injury history, Zielinsky and colleagues [30] found that anhedonia scores were higher in those with prior suicide attempts than in those with a history of non-suicidal self-injury. Depressive symptoms predicted suicidal behavior directly and also via mediation through anhedonia.

Ballard and colleagues [31] carried out a prospective study in order to identify which clinical dimensions (suicidal ideation, loss of interest, anxiety, psychomotor agitation, high-risk behavior) increase before suicidal behavior. Data were collected from the Systematic Treatment Enhancement Program for Bipolar Disorder (STEP-BD) study. All the patients included were affected by bipolar disorders. Ballard et al. compared the participants who attempted suicide or completed suicide ($n = 103$) with patients without suicidal behavior ($n = 427$). The results indicated that patients with suicidal behavior had an elevation of all symptoms, including loss of interest. Moreover, suicidal ideation and loss of interest were highly intense in the months before the suicidal behavior so that they could be considered to be a risk factor for suicidal behavior in bipolar patients.

In a cross-sectional study [12], Xie et al. explored the contribution of anhedonia and avoidance of pain as central factors in influencing the suicidal mind in a cohort of 40 depressed outpatients and 20 healthy control subjects. In the Affective Incentive Delay (AID) task, the High Suicidal Ideation (HIS) group had longer response times (RTs) under the reward condition than under the punishment condition, while the Low Suicidal Ideation (LSI) group and control groups had shorter RTs under the reward condition than under the neutral condition. The LSI group had also shorter RTs under the reward condition than under the punishment condition. Moreover, pain arousal and scores on the Beck Scale for Suicide Ideation (BSS) were negatively associated with differences in RTs between neutral and reward conditions, while pain avoidance and BSS scores were positively associated with differences in RTs between neutral and punishment conditions. Xie et al. concluded that the AID task was the best task for the detection of a hedonic approach to experience and of pain avoidance so that a reduced motivation to experience pleasure and an increased motivation to avoid pain could be considered reliable predictors of suicidal behavior.

In order to explore determinants of suicidal ideation and suicide attempts, Spijker and colleagues [32] carried out a prospective epidemiologic survey in the 2009 Netherlands Mental Health Survey and Incidence Study. They studied 586 adults with ≥2 depressive symptoms (according to the Composite International Diagnostic Interview-CIDI). The results indicated that the rates of suicidal ideation and suicide attempts in the observed population were, respectively, 16.6% and 3.2%. Several clinical factors seemed to be related to an increased risk of suicide: longer duration (13 months) of depression ($p = 0.01$), anhedonia ($p = 0.005$), feeling useless ($p = 0.03$), anxiety ($p < 0.01$), previous suicidal ideation ($p < 0.001$), and access to professional care ($p = 0.05$).

Oei and colleagues [34] conducted a cross-sectional study on 46 patients with depressive symptoms recruited from the Department of Psychiatry at the University Hospital in Utrecht (Netherlands). Using several measures of both suicidal ideation and anhedonia, they found that anhedonia scores were positively associated with suicidal ideation scores. Of the anhedonic patients, 71% had suicidal ideation.

Fawcett and colleagues [16] investigated the possible role of anhedonia in suicidal behavior as a time-related predictor of suicide in major affective disorder, together with other clinical features. In this prospective study of 954 patients affected by major affective disorder, among the nine clinical features studied, the following were correlated with the risk of dying by suicide within 13 months from baseline: anhedonia, panic attacks, severe anxiety, diminished concentration, moderate alcohol abuse, and global insomnia. Long-term suicides (after 13 months from the baseline) were associated with hopelessness and prior suicidal ideation.

3.2. Schizophrenic Spectrum Disorders

Jahn and colleagues [35] studied 162 patients affected by schizophrenia or schizoaffective disorder and found that motivation and pleasure scores as rated by the Clinical Assessment Interview for negative symptoms (CAINS) were not directly associated with recent suicidal ideation. However, motivation and pleasure-related scores moderated the relationship between social role functioning and suicide ideation.

Loas and colleagues [18] investigated the protective nature of negative symptoms by comparing positive and negative symptoms in schizophrenic patients who died by suicide with non-suicidal schizophrenic patients in a prospective study of 150 patients with chronic schizophrenia. They found out that negative symptoms and the deficit syndrome [defined as a subgroup of schizophrenic patients with at least two enduring, primary or idiopathic, negative symptoms (e.g., poverty of speech, restricted affect, diminished emotional range, interests, sense of purpose or social drive) as assessed by the Positive and Negative Syndrome Scale (PANSS) and the subscale of the Brief Psychiatric Rating Scale (BPRS)] were associated with a lower risk of suicide in these patients. The incidence of the deficit syndrome in the suicides (0%) was lower than the incidence in non-suicidal patients (23.5%).

3.3. Post-Traumatic Stress Disorder (PTSD)

Spitzer and colleagues [36] conducted a cross-sectional study in a sample of 373 trauma-exposed psychology undergraduate students to examine the relationship between acquired capability for suicide (ACS) and DSM–5 PTSD symptom clusters. Whereas most PTSD symptom clusters had a negative association with ACS, the anhedonia cluster was positively related to both facets of ACS: fearlessness of the pain involved in dying (FOP) and fearlessness about death (FAD). The relationship between anhedonia and ACS may explain the decreased fear of death and the higher levels of pain tolerance that contribute to lethal suicidal behavior in PTSD patients.

Guina and colleagues [37] studied 480 adults from military medical centers with previous trauma. The PTSD symptoms most strongly associated with suicide attempts were anhedonia, negative beliefs, and recklessness. Suicide attempts were also significantly associated with worse total PTSD symptom severity, childhood physical abuse, the violent death of a loved one, childhood neglect, childhood sexual abuse, substance, alcohol problem, and benzodiazepine prescriptions.

Chen and colleagues [38] analyzed the data from 36,309 U.S. adults (≥18 years) from the National Epidemiologic Survey on Alcohol and Related Conditions-III and found that both PTSD and anhedonia were associated with attempting suicide.

3.4. Other Diagnoses

Hawes et al. [50] explored the different effects of chronic vs. acute anhedonia on suicidal ideation and lifetime suicide attempt history in a prospective study of 395 adult psychiatric outpatient centers in New York City between January 2016 and March 2017. They found out that recent changes in the capacity to experience pleasure was more powerful in predicting near-term suicidal ideation than was chronic anhedonia.

Winer et al. [11] investigated the association between suicidal ideation and anhedonia in a prospective cohort study of 1529 adult psychiatric inpatients with various diagnoses from DSM-IV using the Beck Depression Inventory II. Anhedonia was associated with suicidal ideation at baseline and at the termination of the study. Changes in anhedonia from baseline to termination predicted a change in suicidal ideation, and anhedonia was a predictor of suicidal ideation regardless of cognitive/affective symptoms of depression.

Loas and colleagues [40] studied 122 psychiatric patients hospitalized in the psychiatric unit of the CHU of Amiens between 2010 and 2013. They found that suicidal ideation as measured by the Beck Depression Inventory was associated with anticipatory anhedonia as measured by the Physical Anhedonia Scale (PAS) (but not PAS consummatory anhedonia) and with anhedonia as measured by the BDI, but not with scores on the Temporal Experience of Pleasure Scale (TEPS).

3.5. Attempted Suicides

Yaseen and colleagues [39] conducted a cross-sectional study to evaluate the relationship between suicidal behavior and anhedonia, anxiety, feelings of being trapped, and frightened attachment in 135 adults admitted to the Emergency Room of the Mount Sinai Beth Israel Hospital (New York) for a suicide attempt or with high suicidal risk. All participants reported suicidal ideation in the past month. Suicidal behavior was assessed with the Columbia Suicide-Severity Rating Scale (C-SSRS). The results showed that prior suicidal ideation was significantly associated with anhedonia, anxiety, and feelings of entrapment. Entrapment and anhedonia were independently associated also with the severity of suicidal ideation.

Loas and colleagues [33] examined the correlation between anhedonia and suicide risk in a cross-sectional study of 106 attempted suicides (30 non-depressed and 73 depressed) and 104 normal controls. The participants were evaluated using the PAS and BDI. Depressed attempters were significantly more anhedonic than controls and non-depressed attempters, while no statistically significant difference on the PAS score emerged between healthy subjects and non-depressed attempters.

Loas [13] followed-up for 6.5 years 106 patients who attempted suicide and who were admitted to the Hospital Nord d'Amiens (between September 1993 and August 1996). During the follow-up period, 6.7% of the patients died by suicide. The patients who completed suicide had a significantly lower score on the PAS as compared to the non-suicide group. Thus, this prospective cohort study indicated that a low level of anhedonia was associated with death from suicide.

3.6. Others

In a cross-sectional study, Daghigh et al. [51] tried to replicate findings of the association between anhedonia, suicide ideation ad suicide attempts [19] in an Iranian sample of 404 students at Kashan University (in the center of Iran). In addition to the surprising finding that the Iranian students were more anhedonic than were the American students (more than double), the authors reported that anhedonia was associated with suicidal risk, independently of other symptoms of depression, and also with suicide attempts.

Loas and colleagues [41] found that anhedonia was related to both suicidal ideation and suicide attempts in a population of 557 physicians. Anhedonia mediated the relationship between suicidal ideation and perceived burdensomeness and thwarted belongingness, variables relevant to Joiner's Interpersonal Theory of Suicide [44]. Two different features of anhedonia (lack of satisfaction and loss of energy) were associated with suicidal behavior. Lack of satisfaction had an impact on suicidal ideation, while loss of energy had an impact on suicide attempts.

In a cross-sectional study, Winer and colleagues [19] studied a population of 1122 undergraduate students at a public university in the southern United States and found that anhedonia was associated with suicidal ideation, but not with suicide attempts.

A cross-sectional study by Loas [42] investigated the association between anhedonia, depression, and suicidal behavior in 224 healthy patients (using the PAS and the BDI) and found that anhedonia scores were not associated with depression scores or current suicidal ideation.

4. Discussion

The present review of the literature suggested that findings on anhedonia and suicidal behavior are inconsistent, and it is difficult to propose a theoretical framework that could explain all the research findings. Some studies in this review reported a positive association between the presence of anhedonia and suicidal behavior (high anhedonia scores were associated with suicidal behavior), regardless of the diagnosis of the patients. Other studies found a negative association (low anhedonia scores were associated with suicidal behavior), and a few studies reported no association. The included studies, organized by type of disorder, are summarized in Table 1.

The role of psychiatric diagnosis in the association of anhedonia with suicidal behavior appears to be important. The most consistent association was found for patients with affective disorders (7 of 7 studies reported a significant positive association) and for patients with PTSD (3 of 3 studies reported a positive association). For the two studies of patients with schizophrenia, one found no association (Jahn et al. [35]) and the other found a negative association (Loas et al. [18]). For patients who had attempted suicide (and who were undiagnosed), one study found a positive association [39], one a positive association but only for depressed attempters [33], and one found a negative association [13].

The results are also made complex by the type of suicidal risk studied. Winer et al. [19] reported a positive association between anhedonia and suicidal ideation but not for anhedonia and attempted suicide. A meta-analysis by Ducasse and colleagues [45] confirmed that anhedonia scores are higher among patients with than without current suicidal ideation. That meta-analysis evaluated the results of 15 case-control studies, which included 7347 participants (mean age = 30 yrs.) and compared the results for subjects with current suicidal ideation ($n = 657$) vs. subjects without current suicidal ideation ($n = 6690$). Patients affected by different psychiatric disorders (depression; schizophrenia; personality disorders; substance abuse disorder) and subjects without psychiatric diagnosis were included. The results demonstrated that the group with current suicidal ideation presented higher level of anhedonia vs. the group without suicidal ideation ($p < 0.001$; CI = 0.37–0.79). Moreover, the subgroup analysis conducted for a group of patients with homogenous depression scale scores showed that the association between anhedonia and suicidal ideation was not influenced by depression. Those results suggested that people with suicidal ideation had higher level of anhedonia, independently of the presence of depression. For completed suicides, Ballard et al. [31] reported a positive association, whereas Loas et al. [13] reported a negative association. The results may also be made complex by the high incidence of anhedonia in psychiatric patients, as high as 50% as reported in a study from Silverstone [43].

Why is there an association between suicide and anhedonia? The tendency to avoid emotions experienced as unpleasant can be a maladaptive coping strategy [46], and suicidal ideation could also be an avoidance strategy [47,48]. However, avoiding experiences leads to the attenuation of pleasant emotions and the exacerbation of unpleasant ones [49]. The association between current suicidal ideation and anhedonia may also be related to the interaction between the social component of anhedonia (loss of interest in people) and thwarted belongingness, as described by Joiner's Interpersonal Theory of Suicide [44].

This review had several limitations. The studies differed in sample size, study design, and methodology. There were several different measures of anhedonia used in the various studies, and not all of them may be reliable, valid, and equivalent measures. Furthermore, some of the studies did not accurately diagnose the patients, and we have seen in the present review that psychiatric diagnosis may affect the results of the research. Finally, we respected the choice of some authors to use the generic term of "suicidality" [12,32,39,41] to indicate different aspects of the issue, even if we believe that it could be a source of misunderstanding. A more specific term, such as "suicidal risk," is preferable.

5. Conclusions

The relationship between anhedonia and suicidal behavior is complex. The majority of studies included in our review reported a positive correlation between anhedonia and suicidal risk. The most consistent positive association was found for patients with affective disorders and for patients with PTSD. The positive association was most consistent for suicidal ideation, but less consistent for attempted suicide and completed suicide. However, our review suggests that the assessment of anhedonia may be useful in the evaluation of suicidal risk in depressed patients.

Author Contributions: The main contributions of the individual authors are illustrated as follows: conceptualization, M.P. and L.B.; methodology, L.B.; validation, D.L., L.B. and A.F.; formal analysis, D.L.; investigation, L.B. and F.G.; resources, G.F.; data curation, L.B.; writing—original draft preparation, L.B. and F.G.; writing—review and editing, D.L.; visualization, A.N.; supervision, M.P.; project administration, L.B.

Funding: This research received no external funding.

Conflicts of Interest: The authors declare no conflict of interest.

References

1. World Health Organization. *Preventing Suicide: A Global Imperative*; WHO Press: Geneva, Switzerland, 2014; ISBN 978-924-156-477-9.
2. Jimenez-Trevino, L.; Saiz, P.A.; Corcoran, P.; Garcia-Portilla, M.P.; Buron, P.; Garrido, M.; Bobes, J. The incidence of hospital-treated attempted suicide in Oviedo, Spain. *Crisis* **2012**, *33*, 46–53. [CrossRef] [PubMed]
3. Pompili, M.; Gonda, X.; Serafini, G.; Innamorati, M.; Sher, L.; Amore, M.; Rihmer, Z.; Girardi, P. Epidemiology of suicide in bipolar disorders: A systematic review of the literature. *Bipolar Disord.* **2013**, *15*, 457–490. [CrossRef] [PubMed]
4. Associate Minister of Health. *The New Zealand Suicide Prevention Strategy 2006–2016*; Ministry of Health: Wellington, New Zealand, 2006; ISBN 047-829-995-8.
5. White, J. *Suicide-Related Research in Canada: A Descriptive Overview*; A Background Paper Prepared for the Workshop on Suicide-Related Research; Centre for Suicide Prevention and Centre for Research and Intervention on Suicide and Euthanasia: Montreal, QC, Canada, 2003.
6. World Health Organization. Depression/Suicide. 2002. Available online: http://www.int/health_topics/suicide/en/ (accessed on 12 February 2019).
7. Klonsky, E.D.; May, A.M. Differentiating suicide attempters from suicide ideators: A critical frontier for suicidology research. *Suicide Life Threat. Behav.* **2014**, *44*, 1–5. [CrossRef] [PubMed]
8. Sadock, B.J.; Sadock, V.A.; Ruiz, P. *Kaplan & Sadock's Comprehensive Textbook of Psychiatry*, 10th ed.; Lippincott Williams & Wilkins (LWW): Philadelphia, PA, USA, 2017; ISBN 978-145-110-047-1.
9. Winer, E.S.; Veilleux, J.C.; Ginger, E.J. Development and validation of the specific loss of interest and pleasure scale (SLIPS). *J. Affect. Disord.* **2014**, *152*, 193–201. [CrossRef] [PubMed]
10. Nock, M.K.; Kazdin, A.E. Examination of affective, cognitive, and behavioral factors and suicide-related outcomes in children and young adolescents. *J. Clin. Child Adolesc. Psychol.* **2002**, *31*, 48–58. [CrossRef] [PubMed]
11. Winer, E.S.; Nadorff, M.R.; Ellis, T.E.; Allen, J.G.; Herrera, S.; Salem, T. Anhedonia predicts suicidal ideation in a large psychiatric inpatient sample. *Psychiatry Res.* **2014**, *218*, 124–128. [CrossRef] [PubMed]
12. Xie, W.; Li, H.; Luo, X.; Fu, R.; Ying, X.; Wang, N.; Shi, C. Anhedonia and pain avoidance in the suicidal mind: Behavioral evidence for motivational manifestations of suicidal ideation in patients with major depressive disorder. *J. Clin. Psychol.* **2014**, *70*, 681–692. [CrossRef]
13. Loas, G. Anhedonia and suicide: A 6.5-yr follow-up study of patients hospitalised for a suicide attempt. *Psychol. Rep.* **2007**, *100*, 183–190. [CrossRef]
14. Watson, C.G.; Kucala, T. Anhedonia and death. *Psychol. Rep.* **1978**, *43*, 1120–1122. [CrossRef]
15. Fawcett, J.; Clark, D.C.; Busch, K. Assessing and treating the patient at risk for suicide. *Psychiatr. Ann.* **1993**, *23*, 244–255. [CrossRef]
16. Fawcett, J.; Scheftner, W.A.; Fogg, L.; Clark, D.C.; Young, M.A.; Hedeker, D.; Gibbons, R. Time-related predictors of suicide in major affective disorder. *Am. J. Psychiatry* **1990**, *147*, 1189–1194. [CrossRef] [PubMed]
17. Hall, R.C.; Platt, D.E.; Hall, R.C.W. Suicide risk assessment: A review of risk factors for suicide in 100 patients who made severe suicide attempts. Evaluation of suicide risk in a time of managed care. *Psychosomatics* **1999**, *40*, 18–27. [CrossRef]

18. Loas, G.; Azi, A.; Noisette, C.; Legrand, A.; Yon, V. Fourteen-year prospective follow-up study of positive and negative symptoms in chronic schizophrenic patients dying from suicide compared to other causes of death. *Psychopathology* **2009**, *42*, 185–189. [CrossRef] [PubMed]
19. Winer, E.S.; Drapeau, C.W.; Veilleux, J.C.; Nadorff, M.R. The Association between Anhedonia, Suicidal Ideation, and Suicide Attempts in a Large Student Sample. *Arch. Suicide Res.* **2016**, *20*, 265–272. [CrossRef] [PubMed]
20. Reisch, T.; Seifritz, E.; Esposito, F.; Wiest, R.; Valach, L.; Michel, K. An fMRI study on mental pain and suicidal behavior. *J. Affect. Disord.* **2010**, *126*, 321–325. [CrossRef] [PubMed]
21. Ballard, E.D.; Wills, K.; Lally, N.; Richards, E.M.; Luckenbaugh, D.A.; Walls, T.; Zarate, C.A., Jr. Anhedonia as a clinical correlate of suicidal thoughts in clinical ketamine trials. *J. Affect. Disord.* **2017**, *218*, 195–200. [CrossRef] [PubMed]
22. Loas, G. Anhedonia and Risk of Suicide: An Overview. In *Anhedonia: A Comprehensive Handbook Volume II: 247 Neuropsychiatric and Physical Disorder*; Ritsner, M.S., Ed.; Springer Science + Business Media: Dordrecht, The Netherlands, 2014.
23. Fawcett, J.; Busch, K.A.; Jacobs, D.; Kravitz, H.M.; Fogg, L. Suicide: A four-pathway clinical-biochemical model. *Ann. N. Y. Acad. Sci.* **1997**, *836*, 288–301. [CrossRef] [PubMed]
24. Gard, D.E.; Germans, M.G.; Kring, A.M.; John, O.P. Anticipatory and consummatory components of the experience of pleasure: a scale development study. *J. Res. Personal.* **2006**, *40*, 1086–1102. [CrossRef]
25. Klein, D.F. Depression and anhedonia. In *Anhedonia and Affect Deficit States*; Clark, D.C., Fawcett, J., Eds.; PMA Publishing Corporation: New York, NY, USA, 1987; pp. 1–14.
26. Cipriani, A.; Hawton, K.; Stockton, S.; Geddes, J.R. Lithium in the prevention of suicide in mood disorders: Updated systematic review and meta-analysis. *BMJ* **2013**, *27*, f3646. [CrossRef]
27. Zalsman, G.; Hawton, K.; Wasserman, D.; van Heeringen, K.; Arensman, E.; Sarchiapone, M.; Carli, V.; Höschl, C.; Barzilay, R.; Balazs, J.; et al. Suicide prevention strategies revisited: 10-year systematic review. *Lancet Psychiatry* **2016**, *3*, 646–659. [CrossRef]
28. Hennen, J.; Baldessarini, R.J. Suicidalriskduring treatment with clozapine: A meta-analysis. *Schizophr. Res.* **2005**, *73*, 139–145. [CrossRef]
29. Kessler, R.C.; Berglund, P.; Borges, G.; Nock, M.; Wang, P.S. Trends in suicide ideation, plans, gestures, and attempts in the United States, 1990–1992 to 2001–2003. *JAMA* **2005**, *293*, 2487–2495. [CrossRef]
30. Zielinski, M.J.; Veilleux, J.C.; Winer, E.S.; Nadorff, M.R. A short-term longitudinal examination of the relations between depression, anhedonia, and self-injurious thoughts and behaviors in adults with a history of self-injury. *Compr. Psychiatry* **2017**, *73*, 187–195. [CrossRef]
31. Ballard, E.D.; VandeVoort, J.L.; Luckenbaugh, D.A.; Machado-Vieira, R.; Tohen, M.; Zarate, C.A. Acute risk factors for suicide attempts and death: Prospective findings from the STEP-BD study. *Bipolar Disord.* **2016**, *18*, 363–372. [CrossRef]
32. Spijker, J.; de Graaf, R.; Ten Have, M.; Nolen, W.A.; Speckens, A. Predictors of suicidality in depressive spectrum disorders in the general population: Results of the Netherlands MentalHealth Survey and Incidence Study. *Soc. Psychiatry Psychiatr. Epidemiol.* **2010**, *45*, 513–521. [CrossRef]
33. Loas, G.; Perot, J.M.; Chignague, J.F.; Trespalacios, H.; Delahousse, J. Parasuicide, anhedonia, and depression. *Compr. Psychiatry* **2000**, *41*, 369–372. [CrossRef]
34. Oei, T.I.; Verhoeven, W.M.; Westenberg, H.G.; Zwart, F.M.; van Ree, J.M. Anhedonia, suicide ideation and dexamethasone nonsuppression in depressed patients. *J. Psychiatr. Res.* **1990**, *24*, 25–35. [CrossRef]
35. Jahn, D.R.; Bennett, M.E.; Park, S.G.; Gur, R.E.; Horan, W.P.; Kring, A.M.; Blanchard, J.J. The interactive effects of negative symptoms and social role functioning on suicide ideation in individuals with schizophrenia. *Schizophr. Res.* **2016**, *170*, 271–277. [CrossRef]
36. Spitzer, E.G.; Zuromski, K.L.; Davis, M.T.; Witte, T.K.; Weathers, F. Posttraumatic Stress Disorder Symptom Clusters and Acquired Capability for Suicide: A Reexamination Using DSM-5 Criteria. *Suicide Life Threat. Behav.* **2018**, *48*, 105–115. [CrossRef]
37. Guina, J.; Nahhas, R.W.; Mata, N.; Farnsworth, S. Which Posttraumatic Stress Disorder Symptoms, Trauma Types, and Substances Correlate with Suicide Attempts in Trauma Survivors? *Prim. Care Companion CNS Disord.* **2017**, *19*. [CrossRef]

38. Chen, C.M.; Yoon, Y.H.; Harford, T.C.; Grant, B.F. Dimensionality of DSM-5 posttraumatic stress disorder and its association with suicide attempts: Results from the National Epidemiologic Survey on Alcohol and Related Conditions-III. *Soc. Psychiatry Psychiatr. Epidemiol.* **2017**, *52*, 715–725. [CrossRef] [PubMed]
39. Yaseen, Z.S.; Galynker, I.I.; Briggs, J.; Freed, R.D.; Gabbay, V. Functional domains as correlates of suicidality among psychiatric inpatients. *J. Affect. Disord.* **2016**, *203*, 77–83. [CrossRef] [PubMed]
40. Loas, G.; Dalleau, E.; Lecointe, H.; Yon, V. Relationships between anhedonia, alexithymia, impulsivity, suicidal ideation, recent suicide attempt, C-reactive protein and serum lipid levels among 122 inpatients with mood or anxious disorders. *Psychiatry Res.* **2016**, *246*, 296–302. [CrossRef] [PubMed]
41. Loas, G.; Lefebvre, G.; Rotsaert, M.; Englert, Y. Relationships between anhedonia, suicidal ideation and suicide attempts in a large sample of physicians. *PLoS ONE* **2018**, *13*, e0193619. [CrossRef] [PubMed]
42. Loas, G.; Fremaux, D.; Gayant, C.; Boyer, P. Anhedonia, depression, and suicidal ideation. *Percept. Mot. Ski.* **1995**, *80*, 978. [CrossRef] [PubMed]
43. Silverstone, P. Is anhedonia a good measure of depression? *Acta Psychiatr. Scand.* **1991**, *83*, 249–250. [CrossRef] [PubMed]
44. Van Orden, K.A.; Witte, T.K.; Cukrowicz, K.C.; Braithwaite, S.; Selby, E.A.; Joiner, T.E., Jr. The interpersonal theory of suicide. *Psychol. Rev.* **2010**, *117*, 575–600. [CrossRef] [PubMed]
45. Ducasse, D.; Loas, G.; Dassa, D.; Gramaglia, C.; Zeppegno, P.; Guillaume, S.; Olié, E.; Courtet, P. Anhedonia is associated with suicidal ideation independently of depression: A meta-analysis. *Depress. Anxiety* **2018**, *35*, 382–392. [CrossRef]
46. Hayes, S.C.; Wilson, K.G.; Gifford, E.V.; Follette, V.M.; Strosahl, K. Experimental avoidance and behavioral disorders: A functional dimensional approach to diagnosis and treatment. *J. Consult. Clin. Psychol.* **1996**, *64*, 1152–1168. [CrossRef]
47. Harris, R. *Passez à l'ACT: Pratique de la Thérapie D'acceptation et D'engagement*, 2nd ed.; De Boeck Supérieur: Louvain-la-Neuve, Belgium, 2017; ISBN 978-280-730-849-7.
48. Shneidman, E.S. Suicide as psychache. *J. Nerv. Ment. Dis.* **1993**, *181*, 145–147. [CrossRef]
49. Machell, K.A.; Goodman, F.R.; Kashdan, T.B. Experiential avoidance and well-being: A daily diary analysis. *Cogn. Emot.* **2015**, *29*, 351–359. [CrossRef] [PubMed]
50. Hawes, M.; Galynker, I.; Barzilay, S.; Yaseen, Z.S. Anhedonia and suicidal thoughts and behaviors in psychiatric outpatients: The role of acuity. *Depress. Anxiety* **2018**, *35*, 1218–1227. [CrossRef] [PubMed]
51. Daghigh, A.; Daghigh, V.; Niazi, M.; Nadorff, M.R. The association between anhedonia, suicide ideation, and suicide attempts: A replication in a Persian student sample. *Suicide Life Threat. Behav.* **2018**, *49*, 678–683. [CrossRef] [PubMed]

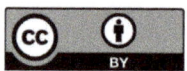

© 2019 by the authors. Licensee MDPI, Basel, Switzerland. This article is an open access article distributed under the terms and conditions of the Creative Commons Attribution (CC BY) license (http://creativecommons.org/licenses/by/4.0/).

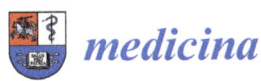

Review

Suicide Risk in Bipolar Disorder: A Brief Review

Peter Dome [1,2,*], **Zoltan Rihmer** [1,2] **and Xenia Gonda** [1,2,3,4]

1. Department of Psychiatry and Psychotherapy, Semmelweis University, Faculty of Medicine, 1125 Budapest, Hungary
2. National Institute of Psychiatry and Addictions, Laboratory for Suicide Research and Prevention, 1135 Budapest, Hungary
3. MTA-SE Neuropsychopharmacology, Neurochemistry Research Group, Hungarian Academy of Sciences, 1089 Budapest, Hungary
4. NAP-2-SE New Antidepressant Target Research Group, Hungarian Brain Research Program, Semmelweis University, 1089 Budapest, Hungary
* Correspondence: dome_peter@yahoo.co.uk; Tel.: +36-30-619-86-20

Received: 19 June 2019; Accepted: 23 July 2019; Published: 24 July 2019

Abstract: Bipolar disorders (BDs) are prevalent mental health illnesses that affect about 1–5% of the total population, have a chronic course and are associated with a markedly elevated premature mortality. One of the contributors for the decreased life expectancy in BD is suicide. Accordingly, the rate of suicide among BD patients is approximately 10–30 times higher than the corresponding rate in the general population. Extant research found that up to 20% of (mostly untreated) BD subjects end their life by suicide, and 20–60% of them attempt suicide at least one in their lifetime. In our paper we briefly recapitulate the current knowledge on the epidemiological aspects of suicide in BD as well as factors associated with suicidal risk in BD. Furthermore, we also discuss concisely the possible means of suicide prevention in BD.

Keywords: bipolar disorder; mood disorders; suicide; suicidal; mortality

1. Introduction

With a lifetime prevalence of 1.3–5.0%, type-I and -II bipolar disorders (BD-I; BD-II) are among the most common psychiatric ailments [1,2]. Patients with BD have poor life expectancies as these patients have a decreased lifespan of about 9–17 years compared with the general population. Furthermore, some studies from different countries (e.g., Denmark and UK) suggest that this mortality gap has become larger over the last decades. Although the largest number of excess death cases in BD may be attributed to natural (e.g., due to cardiovascular diseases or diabetes) and not unnatural causes, suicide is also quite prevalent in the population of subjects with BD [1–5].

At a global scale, approximately 800,000 suicide deaths occur every year (which corresponds to a global suicide rate of 11.4/100,000/year); thus, suicide may be considered a major public health issue [6,7]. Although the great majority (≈90%) of suicide cases occur among subjects with major mental—typically mood–disorders, the majority of patients with mood disorders never become involved in suicidal behaviour. Accordingly, in addition to major mood disorders, other risk factors (including special clinical features of the mental illness as well as some demographic, personality and familial factors) should contribute to suicidality, which therefore should be deemed as a multicausal phenomenon [2,8–10]. Hereinafter, we provide a concise summary of our current knowledge about suicidality in BD based on a review of current literature (mainly review papers, book chapters, meta-analyses, treatment guidelines of international societies, etc.).

2. Epidemiology of Suicidal Behaviour in Bipolar Disorder

Suicidal behaviour is quite frequent among subjects with BD, as up to 4–19% of them ultimately end their life by suicide, while 20–60% of them attempt suicide at least once in their lifetime [2]. In BD, the risk of suicide death is up to 10–30 times higher than that of the general population [2,5,8,10–12]. The estimated annual suicide rate in patients with BD is about 200–400 / 100,000 [8]. BD-associated cases account for about 3–14% of all suicide deaths [13].

It is important to mention that the ratio of suicide attempts to suicide deaths (i.e., the lethality index) is much lower for patients with BD than for the members of the general population (one study, for example, reported that rate as 35:1 and 3:1 for the general population and for BD patients, respectively) [2,8,9]. A possible explanation for this phenomenon may be that BD subjects usually employ more lethal suicide methods compared with members of the general population [2,8,9]. Nevertheless, attempts-to-suicide ratios lower than in the general population are not specific for BD, as it is also observable for instance among patients with schizophrenia or major depressive disorder (MDD) [2,14]. Unsurprisingly, suicidal ideation is also far more frequent in patients with BD (43% past-year prevalence) than in the general population (9.2% life-time prevalence) [7,15].

Though it is indisputable that mood disorders are associated with markedly elevated levels of suicidality, it is hard to pick out from the results of various studies whether there are *relevant* differences in the risk of suicidal behaviour between different kinds of mood disorders. Accordingly, higher, similar or lower levels of suicidality in BD patients compared to MDD patients have also been reported [9,10,16]. In a similar fashion, based on the published information it is hard to disentangle whether any BD subtype (BD-I or BD-II) is associated with a higher level of suicidality than the other [2,8,11,16–19].

It is known that a relatively high proportion (8–55%) of patients with MDD has a history of subthreshold hypomanic symptoms. This so called subthreshold bipolar subgroup of MDD patients differs from MDD patients without subthreshold hypomanic manifestations in several ways. For instance, a wide array of studies demonstrated that subthreshold bipolarity is associated with increased levels of suicidality [20–23].

3. Risk Factors of Suicide in Bipolar Disorder

Several approaches exist to classify risk factors for suicide in BD. One of the most common systems divides risk factors into proximal and distal ones, where proximal (or precipitating) factors are close to suicidal behaviour in time whereas distal factors are rather considered as traits or predispositions and, accordingly, they are enduring [10,24]. Other classifications assign suicide risk factors to conceptual categories (e.g., risk factors associated with genetic or sociodemographic components or illness characteristics or life events) [8,25,26]. Based on different conceptual backgrounds complex models were conceived for the description of the whole process of suicide (e.g., the diathesis-stress model, the bipolar suicidality model, the interpersonal theory of suicide, the three-step theory model or the recently elaborated "neurocognitive model of suicide in the context of bipolar disorders") [10].

In the current paper–without the ambition to be exhaustive–we list and briefly discuss the most relevant risk and protective factors of suicide in BD. In regard to *clinical history*, *previous suicide attempt(s)* is considered as one of the most powerful single predictors of future attempts and suicide death. The *period soon after hospital discharge* may be characterized by extremely high levels of suicidality. This finding draws attention to the importance of avoiding premature discharges and inappropriate follow-ups. In addition, risk of suicide is increased during the *period immediately after hospital admission*. *Frequent and/or great number of prior hospitalizations* are also associated with heightened risk of suicidal self-harming behaviour. *Early age at onset* is also associated with suicidality in BD. The *early years after the diagnosis* represent a high-risk period for suicide. *Comorbidity* with other psychiatric, addictive or severe somatic disorders also increase the risk of all forms of suicidal behaviour. *Rapid-cycling course* and *predominant depressive polarity* during the prior course are also associated with higher risks of self-destructive behaviour. One of the most important determinants of suicidal behavior in BD is the *type/polarity of the current mood episode/state*: pure major depressive episodes and mixed states carry the highest risk, while suicidal behaviour is rarely present in (euphoric) mania, hypomania and during euthymic periods. However, some recent results indicated that there is no elevated risk of suicidal behaviour during mixed state over the risk attributable to its depressed component. Furthermore, these studies suggest that the majority of suicide risk elevation related to having previous mixed states is not an aftermath of the mixed state itself, but can rather be attributed to a depression-predominant course of the disorder. *Longer duration of untreated illness* (i.e., long time lag from the beginning of the affective symptoms until treatment initiation) is also associated with higher hazards of suicidal behaviour. Regarding *sociodemographic factors*, male *gender* is a risk factor for lethal suicides, while, according to some results, female gender is a risk factor for attempts. These gender differences are similar–but weaker–to those observable in the general population; accordingly, in this otherwise high-risk population gender seems not to be a significant predictor for suicidal behaviour). Suicidality is also more frequent among those bipolar subjects who are *divorced*, *unmarried* or *single-parents* or *living in social isolation*. *Age* is a further important sociodemographic factor: BD subjects under 35 years of age and above 75 years of age are at higher risk for engaging in suicide-related behaviours. *Occupational problems and unemployment* also contribute to elevated levels of suicidality. *Adversities in personal history and acute stressors*, such as experiencing sexual or physical abuse and parental loss in childhood or bereavement, breaking the law/criminal conviction and financial disasters are important precipitants of suicidality as well. Some *personality attributes*, for instance impulsive/aggressive traits, hopelessness and pessimism also increase the risk of suicide. Certain types of *affective temperaments* (first and foremost cyclothymic) have also been demonstrated to be associated with more frequent suicidal behaviour in BD. *Family history* of suicide acts and/or major mood disorders are also strong risk factors for suicide in subjects with BD. Some results also suggest that *living in geographical locations where there are large differences in solar insolation between winter and summer* (i.e., near the poles) may be associated with increased risks of attempted suicide in patients with BD-I [2,7,8,10–12,15,17,19,25–34].

4. Protective Factors of Suicide in Bipolar Disorder

In contrast to the above discussed several risk factors for suicide in BD, only a few protective factors have been identified so far [2]. For instance *good family and social support*, *parenthood* and *the use of adaptive coping strategies* seem to have some protective effects. Furthermore, a strong *perceived meaning of life and hyperthymic affective temperament* are also a protective factors [2,10,24,29]. The possible protective role of religiosity has emerged but results are somewhat inconclusive [2,26,35–37]. Last but not least, it is important to note that treatment (and even more so a good response to treatment) is protective against suicide in BD (see also the section "Suicide prevention in bipolar disorder"). In consonance with the fact that treatment may decrease heightened suicidality, it is not surprising that the majority of suicide victims are *untreated* affective disorder patients [8–11,13,38,39].

5. Suicide Prevention in Bipolar Disorder

From a *pharmacological perspective*, *lithium* seems to possess the greatest suicide-preventive potential in patients with BD. Intriguingly, the suicide protective effect of lithium is not confined to bipolar patients as it has also been demonstrated among patients with MDD (it is not surprising since, as we have discussed it previously, a considerable proportion of "unipolar" MDD patients have subthreshold bipolar features) [5,8,15,40–42]. Overall, compared to placebo, lithium appears to decrease the risk of suicide by more than 60% in mood disorders [8,40,42]. Some results suggest that lithium is protective against suicide, albeit in a decreased manner, even in those BD patients who are moderate/poor responders to the phase-prophylactic effect of it. This finding may suggest that in the case of lithium non-response in a patient who is at high risk for suicide, instead of switching lithium to another mood stabilizer, the clinician should retain lithium (even in a lower dose) and combine it with another mood stabilizer [1,41].

A solid suicide-protective effect related to the administration of *anticonvulsant-type mood stabilizers* (e.g., valproic acid, carbamazepine, lamotrigine) to BD patients has not been proven so far. On the other hand, the concern of the FDA about the potential for an increased risk of suicidality associated with anticonvulsants seems not to be applicable to patients with BD (i.e., in this population the use of these agents is not associated with increased levels of suicidality). According to our current knowledge, in regard to suicide prevention lithium is superior than these agents [2,8,15,41,43,44].

The role of *antidepressants* (ADs) in suicide prevention in individuals with BD seems to be negligible, and, in fact, concerns have been raised that administration of ADs may increase suicidality in BD. It is remarkable that findings are also inconsistent regarding the ability of ADs to prevent suicides in patients with MDD. AD monotherapy should be avoided in BD [2,8,15,41].

Considering their increasing use in BD for instance as maintenance treatment, it is justifiable to ask whether (atypical) *antipsychotics* have any beneficial effects on suicidal behaviour in BD. Unfortunately, there are no high-quality data to answer this question at present, so further studies should elucidate whether treatment with antipsychotics has any benefits in this respect [2,8,15,41].

Ketamin as a possible antidepressant agent has mainly been tested in patients with MDD and only a few studies have been conducted among patients with bipolar depression. According to the results of these small proof-of-concept investigations, ketamin shows similar antidepressive efficacy in bipolar as in unipolar depression. In line with its possible efficacy, ketamin is recommended by the clinical guideline of International College of Neuropsychopharmacology (CINP) for the treatment of bipolar depression, but only as a fourth-line agent and in combination with a mood stabilizer. Similarly, until now, the antisuicidal activity of ketamine was assessed mainly in MDD patients and only a small number of investigations have been conducted in BD patients. These have mainly positive outcomes, but further studies are needed to reveal whether ketamin has a similar antisuicidal effect in BD than in MDD [45–51].

It is well-known that *electroconvulsive therapy* (ECT) shows a similar efficacy in the treatment of depressive episodes in MDD and BPD (and some studies even found it more effective against bipolar than unipolar depression). In line with its antidepressive effects, ECT is also considered as an effective antisuicidal treatment modality, and it has been recently demonstrated that it is superior in this regard to psychopharmacons both in unipolar and bipolar depression (and its antisuicidal efficacy is comparable to the efficacy of psychopharmacons in bipolar mixed states and mania) [2,8,41,52,53].

Unfortunately, only a small number of studies have investigated up to now the efficacy of specific (e.g., dialectical behavior therapy, cognitive-behavioural therapy, interpersonal and social rhythm therapy) or unspecific (e.g., psychoeducation) *psychosocial interventions* against suicide among BD patients. Nonetheless, results of the few existing studies are promising [2,8,54–58].

6. Summary and Clinical Implications

BD is a relatively common psychiatric disorder that is associated with increased mortality due to both natural and unnatural causes. Accordingly, the risk of suicide is highly elevated in this patient population. Because of this, a thorough assessment of suicide risk should take place at all clinical visits. This clinical assessment should include, *inter alia*, the comprehensive examination of the mental state, and the inquiry about the existence and features of current suicidal intents (e.g., duration and intensity), the methods intended to be used, the access to means (e.g., weapons) as well as the compliance to prescribed medications. In addition, it is essential to gain information about previous suicidality. Whenever possible, hetero-anamnestic data should be gathered as well. The management of suicidal behaviour in patients with BD represents a clinical challenge. Appropriate long-term treatment of the disorder seems to be associated with the reduction of suicidality. Furthermore, in acutely suicidal patients the removal of access to obvious means for suicide is essential and, in severe cases, hospitalization may be justifiable as well. Prevention strategies should include the provision of psychoeducation (for example, via information leaflets and/or by the members of the health care staff) to the patients, as well as to relatives and friends, in order that they become able to recognize the warning signs of suicidal behaviour, be aware of the risk periods and the importance of adherence to treatment, avoid isolation and call for help in emergency situations. A written list of sources of support which are available during a suicidal crisis may also be helpful [2,10,15,59].

Conflicts of Interest: The authors declare no conflict of interest.

References

1. Rihmer, Z.; Dome, P. Suicide and Bipolar Disorder. In *Bipolar Depression: Molecular Neurobiology, Clinical Diagnosis, and Pharmacotherapy*, 2nd ed.; Zarate, C.A.J.; Manji, H.K., Eds.; Springer: Bern, Switzerland, 2017.
2. Rihmer, Z.; Gonda, X.; Döme, P. The Assessment and Management of SuicideRrisk in Bipolar Disorder. In *The Treatment of Bipolar Disorder: Integrative Clinical Strategies and Future Directions*; Carvalho, A.F., Vieta, E., Eds.; Oxford University Press: Oxford, UK, 2017.
3. Staudt Hansen, P.; Frahm Laursen, M.; Grontved, S.; Puggard Vogt Straszek, S.; Licht, R.W.; Nielsen, R.E. Increasing mortality gap for patients diagnosed with bipolar disorder—A nationwide study with 20 years of follow-up. *Bipolar Disord.* **2019**, *21*, 270–275. [CrossRef] [PubMed]
4. Hayes, J.F.; Marston, L.; Walters, K.; King, M.B.; Osborn, D.P.J. Mortality gap for people with bipolar disorder and schizophrenia: UK-based cohort study 2000–2014. *Br. J. Psychiatry* **2017**, *211*, 175–181. [CrossRef] [PubMed]
5. Bauer, M.; Andreassen, O.A.; Geddes, J.R.; Vedel Kessing, L.; Lewitzka, U.; Schulze, T.G.; Vieta, E. Areas of uncertainties and unmet needs in bipolar disorders: Clinical and research perspectives. *Lancet Psychiatry* **2018**, *5*, 930–939. [CrossRef]
6. World Health Organization. *Preventing Suicide: A Global Imperative*; WHO Press: Geneva, Switzerland, 2014.
7. Turecki, G.; Brent, D.A. Suicide and suicidal behaviour. *Lancet* **2016**, *387*, 1227–1239. [CrossRef]
8. Plans, L.; Barrot, C.; Nieto, E.; Rios, J.; Schulze, T.G.; Papiol, S.; Mitjans, M.; Vieta, E.; Benabarre, A. Association between completed suicide and bipolar disorder: A systematic review of the literature. *J. Affect. Disord.* **2019**, *242*, 111–122. [CrossRef] [PubMed]
9. Rihmer, Z.; Döme, P. Major Mood Disorders and Suicidal Behavior. In *The International Handbook of Suicide Prevention: Research, Policy and Practice*; O'Connor, R.C., Pirkis, J., Eds.; John Wiley and Sons, Ltd.: Chichester, UK, 2016.
10. Malhi, G.S.; Outhred, T.; Das, P.; Morris, G.; Hamilton, A.; Mannie, Z. Modeling suicide in bipolar disorders. *Bipolar Disord.* **2018**, *20*, 334–348. [CrossRef] [PubMed]
11. Vieta, E.; Berk, M.; Schulze, T.G.; Carvalho, A.F.; Suppes, T.; Calabrese, J.R.; Gao, K.; Miskowiak, K.W.; Grande, I. Bipolar disorders. *Nat. Rev. Dis. Primers* **2018**, *4*, 18008. [CrossRef]
12. Pompili, M.; Gonda, X.; Serafini, G.; Innamorati, M.; Sher, L.; Amore, M.; Rihmer, Z.; Girardi, P. Epidemiology of suicide in bipolar disorders: A systematic review of the literature. *Bipolar Disord.* **2013**, *15*, 457–490. [CrossRef]
13. Schaffer, A.; Isometsa, E.T.; Tondo, L.; Moreno, D.H.; Sinyor, M.; Kessing, L.V.; Turecki, G.; Weizman, A.; Azorin, J.-M.; Ha, K.; et al. Epidemiology, neurobiology and pharmacological interventions related to suicide deaths and suicide attempts in bipolar disorder: Part I of a report of the International Society for Bipolar Disorders Task Force on Suicide in Bipolar Disorder. *Aust. N. Z. J. Psychiatry* **2015**, *49*, 785–802. [CrossRef]
14. Desîlets, A.; Labossière, M.; McGirr, A.; Turecki, G. Schizophrenia, Other Psychotic Disorders, and Suicidal Behavior. In *The International Handbook of Suicide Prevention*; O'Connor, R.C., Pirkis, J., Eds.; John Wiley & Sons, Ltd.: Chichester, UK, 2016.
15. Yatham, L.N.; Kennedy, S.H.; Parikh, S.V.; Schaffer, A.; Bond, D.J.; Frey, B.N.; Sharma, V.; I Goldstein, B.; Rej, S.; Beaulieu, S.; et al. Canadian Network for Mood and Anxiety Treatments (CANMAT) and International Society for Bipolar Disorders (ISBD) 2018 guidelines for the management of patients with bipolar disorder. *Bipolar Disord.* **2018**, *20*, 97–170. [CrossRef]
16. Isometsa, E. Suicidal behaviour in mood disorders—Who, when, and why? *Can. J. Psychiatry* **2014**, *59*, 120–130. [CrossRef] [PubMed]
17. Hansson, C.; Joas, E.; Palsson, E.; Hawton, K.; Runeson, B.; Landen, M. Risk factors for suicide in bipolar disorder: A cohort study of 12,850 patients. *Acta Psychiatry Scand.* **2018**, *138*, 456–463. [CrossRef] [PubMed]

18. Tondo, L.; Pompili, M.; Forte, A.; Baldessarini, R.J. Suicide attempts in bipolar disorders: Comprehensive review of 101 reports. *Acta Psychiatry Scand.* **2016**, *133*, 174–186. [CrossRef] [PubMed]
19. Schaffer, A.; Isometsa, E.T.; Tondo, L.; Moreno, D.H.; Turecki, G.; Reis, C.; Cassidy, F.; Sinyor, M.; Azorin, J.-M.; Kessing, L.V.; et al. International Society for Bipolar Disorders Task Force on Suicide: Meta-analyses and meta-regression of correlates of suicide attempts and suicide deaths in bipolar disorder. *Bipolar Disord.* **2015**, *17*, 1–16. [CrossRef] [PubMed]
20. Choi, K.W.; Na, E.J.; Hong, J.P.; Cho, M.J.; Fava, M.; Mischoulon, D.; Jeon, H.J. Comparison of suicide attempts in individuals with major depressive disorder with and without history of subthreshold hypomania: A nationwide community sample of Korean adults. *J. Affect. Disord.* **2019**, *248*, 18–25. [CrossRef] [PubMed]
21. Park, Y.M.; Lee, B.H. Treatment response in relation to subthreshold bipolarity in patients with major depressive disorder receiving antidepressant monotherapy: A post hoc data analysis (KOMDD study). *Neuropsychiatr. Dis. Treat.* **2016**, *12*, 1221–1227. [CrossRef]
22. Koirala, P.; Hu, B.; Altinay, M.; Li, M.; DiVita, A.L.; Bryant, K.A.; Karne, H.S.; Fiedorowicz, J.G.; Anan, A. Sub-threshold bipolar disorder in medication-free young subjects with major depression: Clinical characteristics and antidepressant treatment response. *J. Psychiatr. Res.* **2019**, *110*, 1–8. [CrossRef]
23. Dome, P.; Gonda, X.; Rihmer, Z. Effects of smoking on health outcomes in bipolar disorder with a special focus on suicidal behavior. *Neuropsychiatry* **2012**, *2*, 429–441. [CrossRef]
24. Latalova, K.; Kamaradova, D.; Prasko, J. Suicide in bipolar disorder: A review. *Psychiatr. Danub.* **2014**, *26*, 108–114.
25. Gonda, X.; Pompili, M.; Serafini, G.; Montebovi, F.; Campi, S.; Dome, P.; Duleba, T.; Girardi, P.; Rihmer, Z. Suicidal behavior in bipolar disorder: Epidemiology, characteristics and major risk factors. *J. Affect. Disord.* **2012**, *143*, 16–26. [CrossRef]
26. Da Silva Costa, L.; Alencar, A.P.; Nascimento Neto, P.J.; dos Santos Mdo, S.; da Silva, C.G.; Pinheiro Sde, F.; Silveira, R.T.; Bianco, B.A.V.; Junior, R.F.F.P.; De Lima, M.A.P.; et al. Risk factors for suicide in bipolar disorder: A systematic review. *J. Affect. Disord.* **2015**, *170*, 237–254. [CrossRef] [PubMed]
27. Michaels, M.S.; Balthrop, T.; Pulido, A.; Rudd, M.D.; Joiner, T.E. Is the Higher Number of Suicide Attempts in Bipolar Disorder vs. Major Depressive Disorder Attributable to Illness Severity? *Arch. Suicide Res.* **2018**, *22*, 46–56. [CrossRef] [PubMed]
28. Pallaskorpi, S.; Suominen, K.; Ketokivi, M.; Valtonen, H.; Arvilommi, P.; Mantere, O.; Leppämäki, S.; Isometsä, E. Incidence and predictors of suicide attempts in bipolar I and II disorders: A 5-year follow-up study. *Bipolar Disord.* **2017**, *19*, 13–22. [CrossRef] [PubMed]
29. Vazquez, G.H.; Gonda, X.; Lolich, M.; Tondo, L.; Baldessarini, R.J. Suicidal Risk and Affective Temperaments, Evaluated with the TEMPS-A Scale: A Systematic Review. *Harv. Rev. Psychiatry* **2018**, *26*, 8–18. [CrossRef] [PubMed]
30. Persons, J.E.; Coryell, W.H.; Solomon, D.A.; Keller, M.B.; Endicott, J.; Fiedorowicz, J.G. Mixed state and suicide: Is the effect of mixed state on suicidal behavior more than the sum of its parts? *Bipolar Disord.* **2018**, *20*, 35–41. [CrossRef] [PubMed]
31. Fiedorowicz, J.G.; Persons, J.E.; Assari, S.; Ostacher, M.J.; Zandi, P.; Wang, P.W.; Thase, M.E.; Frye, M.A.; Coryell, W. Depressive symptoms carry an increased risk for suicidal ideation and behavior in bipolar disorder without any additional contribution of mixed symptoms. *J. Affect. Disord.* **2019**, *246*, 775–782. [CrossRef] [PubMed]
32. Tidemalm, D.; Haglund, A.; Karanti, A.; Landen, M.; Runeson, B. Attempted suicide in bipolar disorder: Risk factors in a cohort of 6086 patients. *PLoS ONE* **2014**, *9*, e94097. [CrossRef]
33. Manchia, M.; Hajek, T.; O'Donovan, C.; Deiana, V.; Chillotti, C.; Ruzickova, M.; Del Zompo, M.; Alda, M. Genetic risk of suicidal behavior in bipolar spectrum disorder: Analysis of 737 pedigrees. *Bipolar Disord.* **2013**, *15*, 496–506. [CrossRef]
34. Bauer, M.; Glenn, T.; Alda, M.; Andreassen, O.A.; Angelopoulos, E.; Ardau, R.; Ayhan, Y.; Baethge, C.; Bauer, R.; Baune, B.T.; et al. Association between solar insolation and a history of suicide attempts in bipolar I disorder. *J. Psychiatr. Res.* **2019**, *113*, 1–9. [CrossRef]
35. Caribe, A.C.; Studart, P.; Bezerra-Filho, S.; Brietzke, E.; Nunes Noto, M.; Vianna-Sulzbach, M.; Kapczinski, F.; Neves, F.S.; Corrêa, H.; Miranda-Scippa, A. Is religiosity a protective factor against suicidal behavior in bipolar I outpatients? *J. Affect. Disord.* **2015**, *186*, 156–161. [CrossRef]

36. Gearing, R.E.; Alonzo, D. Religion and Suicide: New Findings. *J. Relig. Health* **2018**, *57*, 2478–2499. [CrossRef] [PubMed]
37. Schaffer, A.; Isometsa, E.T.; Azorin, J.M.; Cassidy, F.; Goldstein, T.; Rihmer, Z.; Sinyor, M.; Tondo, L.; Moreno, D.H.; Turecki, G.; et al. A review of factors associated with greater likelihood of suicide attempts and suicide deaths in bipolar disorder: Part II of a report of the International Society for Bipolar Disorders Task Force on Suicide in Bipolar Disorder. *Aust. N. Z. J. Psychiatry* **2015**, *49*, 1006–1020. [CrossRef] [PubMed]
38. Novick, D.M.; Swartz, H.A.; Frank, E. Suicide attempts in bipolar I and bipolar II disorder: A review and meta-analysis of the evidence. *Bipolar Disord.* **2010**, *12*, 1–9. [CrossRef] [PubMed]
39. Angst, J.; Sellaro, R.; Angst, F. Long-term outcome and mortality of treated versus untreated bipolar and depressed patients: A preliminary report. *Int. J. Psychiatry Clin. Pract.* **1998**, *2*, 115–119. [CrossRef] [PubMed]
40. Smith, K.A.; Cipriani, A. Lithium and suicide in mood disorders: Updated meta-review of the scientific literature. *Bipolar Disord.* **2017**, *19*, 575–586. [CrossRef] [PubMed]
41. Tondo, L.; Baldessarini, R.J. Antisuicidal Effects in Mood Disorders: Are They Unique to Lithium? *Pharmacopsychiatry* **2018**, *51*, 177–188. [CrossRef]
42. Cipriani, A.; Hawton, K.; Stockton, S.; Geddes, J.R. Lithium in the prevention of suicide in mood disorders: Updated systematic review and meta-analysis. *BMJ* **2013**, *346*, f3646. [CrossRef] [PubMed]
43. Chen, T.Y.; Kamali, M.; Chu, C.S.; Yeh, C.B.; Huang, S.Y.; Mao, W.C.; Lin, P.-Y.; Chen, Y.-W.; Tseng, P.-T.; Hsu, C.-Y. Divalproex and its effect on suicide risk in bipolar disorder: A systematic review and meta-analysis of multinational observational studies. *J. Affect. Disord.* **2019**, *245*, 812–818. [CrossRef]
44. Caley, C.F.; Perriello, E.; Golden, J. Antiepileptic drugs and suicide-related outcomes in bipolar disorder: A descriptive review of published data. *Ment. Health Clin.* **2018**, *8*, 138–147. [CrossRef]
45. Alberich, S.; Martinez-Cengotitabengoa, M.; Lopez, P.; Zorrilla, I.; Nunez, N.; Vieta, E.; González-Pinto, A. Efficacy and safety of ketamine in bipolar depression: A systematic review. *Rev. Psiquiatr. Salud Ment.* **2017**, *10*, 104–112. [CrossRef]
46. Lopez-Diaz, A.; Fernandez-Gonzalez, J.L.; Lujan-Jimenez, J.E.; Galiano-Rus, S.; Gutierrez-Rojas, L. Use of repeated intravenous ketamine therapy in treatment-resistant bipolar depression with suicidal behaviour: A case report from Spain. *Ther. Adv. Psychopharmacol.* **2017**, *7*, 137–140. [CrossRef] [PubMed]
47. Andrade, C. Ketamine for Depression, 6: Effects on Suicidal Ideation and Possible Use as Crisis Intervention in Patients at Suicide Risk. *J. Clin. Psychiatry* **2018**, *79*. [CrossRef] [PubMed]
48. Grunebaum, M.F.; Ellis, S.P.; Keilp, J.G.; Moitra, V.K.; Cooper, T.B.; Marver, J.E.; Burke, A.K.; Milak, M.S.; Sublette, M.E.; Oquendo, M.A.; et al. Ketamine versus midazolam in bipolar depression with suicidal thoughts: A pilot midazolam-controlled randomized clinical trial. *Bipolar Disord.* **2017**, *19*, 176–183. [CrossRef] [PubMed]
49. Sanacora, G.; Katz, R. Ketamine: A Review for Clinicians. *Focus* **2018**, *16*, 243–250. [CrossRef]
50. Sanches, M.; Quevedo, J.; Soares, J.C. Treatment Resistance in Bipolar Disorders. In *Treatment Resistance in Psychiatry*; Kim, Y.-K., Ed.; Springer Nature: Singapore, 2019.
51. Fountoulakis, K.N.; Grunze, H.; Vieta, E.; Young, A.; Yatham, L.; Blier, P.; Kasper, S.; Moeller, H.J. The International College of Neuro-Psychopharmacology (CINP) Treatment Guidelines for Bipolar Disorder in Adults (CINP-BD-2017), Part 3: The Clinical Guidelines. *Int. J. Neuropsychopharmacol.* **2017**, *20*, 180–195. [CrossRef] [PubMed]
52. Liang, C.S.; Chung, C.H.; Ho, P.S.; Tsai, C.K.; Chien, W.C. Superior anti-suicidal effects of electroconvulsive therapy in unipolar disorder and bipolar depression. *Bipolar Disord.* **2018**, *20*, 539–546. [CrossRef] [PubMed]
53. Bahji, A.; Hawken, E.R.; Sepehry, A.A.; Cabrera, C.A.; Vazquez, G. ECT beyond unipolar major depression: Systematic review and meta-analysis of electroconvulsive therapy in bipolar depression. *Acta Psychiatr. Scand.* **2019**, *139*, 214–226. [CrossRef] [PubMed]
54. Mendez-Bustos, P.; Calati, R.; Rubio-Ramirez, F.; Olie, E.; Courtet, P.; Lopez-Castroman, J. Effectiveness of Psychotherapy on Suicidal Risk: A Systematic Review of Observational Studies. *Front. Psychol.* **2019**, *10*, 277. [CrossRef]
55. Inder, M.L.; Crowe, M.T.; Luty, S.E.; Carter, J.D.; Moor, S.; Frampton, C.M.; Joyce, P.R. Prospective rates of suicide attempts and nonsuicidal self-injury by young people with bipolar disorder participating in a psychotherapy study. *Aust. N. Z. J. Psychiatry* **2016**, *50*, 167–173. [CrossRef]

56. Rucci, P.; Frank, E.; Kostelnik, B.; Fagiolini, A.; Mallinger, A.G.; Swartz, H.A.; Thase, M.E.; Siegel, L.; Wilson, D.; Kupfer, D.J. Suicide attempts in patients with bipolar I disorder during acute and maintenance phases of intensive treatment with pharmacotherapy and adjunctive psychotherapy. *Am. J. Psychiatry* **2002**, *159*, 1160–1164. [CrossRef]
57. Weinstein, S.M.; Cruz, R.A.; Isaia, A.R.; Peters, A.T.; West, A.E. Child- and Family-Focused Cognitive Behavioral Therapy for Pediatric Bipolar Disorder: Applications for Suicide Prevention. *Suicide Life-Threat Behav.* **2018**, *48*, 797–811. [CrossRef] [PubMed]
58. Goldstein, T.R.; Fersch-Podrat, R.K.; Rivera, M.; Axelson, D.A.; Merranko, J.; Yu, H.; Brent, D.A.; Birmaher, B. Dialectical behavior therapy for adolescents with bipolar disorder: Results from a pilot randomized trial. *J. Child Adolesc. Psychopharmacol.* **2015**, *25*, 140–149. [CrossRef] [PubMed]
59. Wasserman, D.; Rihmer, Z.; Rujescu, D.; Sarchiapone, M.; Sokolowski, M.; Titelman, D.; Zalsman, G.; Zemishlany, Z.; Carli, V. The European Psychiatric Association (EPA) guidance on suicide treatment and prevention. *Eur. Psychiatry* **2012**, *27*, 129–141. [CrossRef] [PubMed]

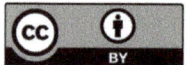

© 2019 by the authors. Licensee MDPI, Basel, Switzerland. This article is an open access article distributed under the terms and conditions of the Creative Commons Attribution (CC BY) license (http://creativecommons.org/licenses/by/4.0/).

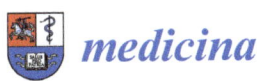

Review
Suicide in Schizophrenia: An Educational Overview

Leo Sher [1,2,*] and René S. Kahn [1,2]

1 James J. Peters Veterans' Administration Medical Center, Bronx, New York, NY 10468, USA
2 Icahn School of Medicine at Mount Sinai, New York, NY 10029, USA
* Correspondence: Leo.Sher@mssm.edu; Tel.: +1-718-584-9000 (ext. 6821)

Received: 16 June 2019; Accepted: 7 July 2019; Published: 10 July 2019

Abstract: Suicide is an important public health problem. The most frequent psychiatric illnesses associated with suicide or severe suicide attempt are mood and psychotic disorders. The purpose of this paper is to provide an educational overview of suicidal behavior in individuals with schizophrenia. A lifetime suicide rate in individuals with schizophrenia is approximately 10%. Suicide is the largest contributor to the decreased life expectancy in individuals with schizophrenia. Demographic and psychosocial factors that increase a risk of suicide in individuals with schizophrenia include younger age, being male, being unmarried, living alone, being unemployed, being intelligent, being well-educated, good premorbid adjustment or functioning, having high personal expectations and hopes, having an understanding that life's expectations and hopes are not likely to be met, having had recent (i.e., within past 3 months) life events, having poor work functioning, and having access to lethal means, such as firearms. Throughout the first decade of their disorder, patients with schizophrenia are at substantially elevated suicide risk, although they continue to be at elevated suicide risk during their lives with times of worsening or improvement. Having awareness of symptoms, especially, awareness of delusions, anhedonia, asociality, and blunted affect, having a negative feeling about, or non-adherence with, treatment are associated with greater suicide risk in patients with schizophrenia. Comorbid depression and a history of suicidal behavior are important contributors to suicide risk in patients with schizophrenia. The only reliable protective factor for suicide in patients with schizophrenia is provision of and compliance with comprehensive treatment. Prevention of suicidal behavior in schizophrenia should include recognizing patients at risk, delivering the best possible therapy for psychotic symptoms, and managing comorbid depression and substance misuse.

Keywords: suicide; schizophrenia; antipsychotics; depression

1. Suicide as a Medical and Social Problem

Suicide is an important public health problem [1,2]. According to the World health Organization (WHO), each year, about one million people die by suicide across the world [1]. It implies that every 40 s, an individual dies by suicide someplace on the globe and many more people make non-lethal suicide attempts. It has been proposed that the number of persons who make non-lethal suicide attempts is about 10–15 times the amount of people who die by suicide. Deaths by suicide and non-lethal suicide attempts greatly affect families, communities, and societies. In the United States, the expenses of managing suicide attempters and examining deaths by suicide have been assessed as being $190 million per year [3]. A recent study showed that non-lethal suicide attempts are associated with decreased life span [4]. It is worth noting that this study found that most additional deaths are attributable to physical/medical conditions.

Rates of suicide death are very significant in many countries across the world [1]. A report issued in November 2018 by the United States Centers for Disease Control and Prevention indicates that from 1999 through 2017, the age-adjusted rate of suicide in the United States rose 33% from 10.5 to 14.0 per 100,000 [5]. It is possible that suicide rates are underestimated. A lot of suicide deaths may be wrongly recorded as 'unnatural' or 'undetermined' deaths. Actual suicide rates may well be 10%–50% higher than reported.

Globally, men die by suicide 3–7 times more often than women [1,6]. The sex dissimilarities in suicide rates are particularly substantial in Eastern European nations [1,6]. In the United States, in 2017, the age-adjusted suicide rate for men (22.4 per 100,000) was 3.67 times larger than for women (6.1 per 100,000) [5].

Studies in the U.S. suggest that more than 90% of victims of suicide have a psychiatric disorder [2,7–9]. Furthermore, most people who attempt suicide have a psychiatric disorder. The most frequent psychiatric illnesses associated with suicide or severe suicide attempt are mood and psychotic disorders [2,7–10]. A 5-year follow-up study of 1065 patients with psychotic disorders conducted by the World Health Organization (WHO) found that "the risk for suicide in schizophrenia is as great, if not greater, than the risk of suicide associated with affective disorders" [11]. Alcohol and drug abuse, anxiety and personality disorders are also associated with an elevated suicide risk [12–15].

Medical disorders, particularly illnesses associated with chronic pain, significantly increase suicide risk [16–20]. While many deaths due to opioid overdoses are accidental, an increasing amount of data indicates that the presence of pain plays a role in the decision to end life via opioid overdoses [19]. Neurological conditions such as stroke, epilepsy, head injury, or Huntington's disease also confer greater suicide risk [20,21]. Obstacles to preventing suicidal behavior include inadequate rates of detection of persons with psychiatric illnesses, insufficient dissemination of evidence-based methods among community providers, and enormous complexity in detecting imminent suicide risk, even in persons who are being cared for psychiatric conditions [22,23].

Adolescence is a period of transition from childhood to adulthood and also, a time of increased vulnerability to psychiatric disorders including psychotic disorders [24]. A systematic review suggests that the number of adversities or negative life events experienced by adolescents appear to have a positive dose–response relationship with youth suicidal behavior [25]. Hence, traumatic experiences during adolescence may contribute to the pathophysiology of both psychotic disorders and suicidal behavior.

The purpose of this paper is to provide an educational overview of suicidal behavior in individuals with schizophrenia. Most literature searches were performed using the PubMed database.

2. Epidemiology of Suicidal Behavior in Schizophrenia

As early as 1911, E. Bleuler characterized "the suicidal drive" as the "most serious of all schizophrenic symptoms" [26]. In 1919, Kraepelin stated that suicide happened in both acute and chronic stages of schizophrenia [27]. In 1939, before contemporary treatments became available, Rennie [28] observed that 11 percent of 500 patients with schizophrenia had died by suicide throughout a 20-year follow-up period.

Contemporary research studies indicate that a lifetime rate of suicide in individuals with schizophrenia is between 4% and 13%, while the modal rate is about 10% [29]. The reported rates of suicide attempts in patients with schizophrenia vary between from 18% to 55% [29–31].

Considerable evidence suggests that schizophrenia decreases the longevity by about 10 years [32]. Suicide is the largest contributor to the decreased life expectancy in individuals with schizophrenia. Recognition of suicide risk factors in patients with schizophrenia is vital in order to enhance patient treatment and advance approaches to decrease the incidence of suicide in patients with schizophrenia.

3. Demographic and Psychosocial Risk Factors

Studies and observations suggest that the following demographic and psychosocial factors increase the risk of suicide in individuals with schizophrenia [10,29,33–36]:

- Younger age
- Being male

- Being unmarried
- Living alone
- Being unemployed
- Being intelligent
- Being well-educated
- Good premorbid adjustment or functioning
- Having high personal expectations and hopes
- Having an understanding that life's expectations and hopes are not likely to be met
- Having had recent (i.e., within past 3 months) life events
- Having poor work functioning
- Having access to lethal means, such as firearms

Studies have demonstrated that suicidal behavior takes place when patients with schizophrenia are younger than age 45 years [37–39]. However, this association is probably more related to the onset of schizophrenia than to age itself.

Similar to the general population and patients with other psychiatric disorders, males with schizophrenia die by suicide more frequently than females with schizophrenia, but the gender difference among suicide victims with schizophrenia is considerably less (60% vs. 40%) [40–42]. Unlike the general population in which females usually make more non-lethal suicide acts than do men, rates of suicide attempts among individuals with schizophrenia have not been found to differ by gender [42–44].

Being single and being unemployed are suicide risk factors for individuals with schizophrenia [29,33,34,42,45]. Some researchers believe that there is a problem with interpreting these findings because most persons with schizophrenia are single and unemployed.

4. Risk Factors Related to Symptomatology and the Course of Illness

Throughout the first decade of their disorder, patients with schizophrenia are at substantially elevated suicide risk, although they continue to be at elevated suicide risk during their lives, with times of worsening or improvement [33,42,46]. Excess mortality due to suicide during the 40-year follow up of 200 patients with schizophrenia was as follows: 44 percent of the patients with schizophrenia who died by suicide committed suicide during the first decade of observation, 22 percent during the second decade, and another 22 percent during the third decade [47].

Studies indicate that suicide risk is significantly elevated during the first psychotic break [29,46,48–50]. Research of first-episode patients usually has higher estimations of suicide rates than studies with lengthier follow up periods. It has been noted that during early stages of schizophrenia, limited suicidal ideation may quickly intensify to a suicide attempt. A delay in getting psychiatric treatment may substantially contribute to elevated suicide risk early in the course of schizophrenia. Other suicide risk factors early in the course of schizophrenia include earlier age of the onset of psychotic symptoms, female sex, suicidal plans, a history of suicide attempt, seriousness of psychiatric pathology, a history of emotional trauma, and decent insight. Suicidality during the first psychotic episode is associated with a good understanding of the situation and beliefs about bad outcomes for psychotic conditions.

Having had an earlier age of onset, being in an early part of the course of illness, having awareness of symptoms, especially, awareness of delusions, anhedonia, asociality, and blunted affect, having a negative feeling about, or non-adherence with, treatment are associated with greater suicide risk in patients with schizophrenia [33,51–53]. In addition, a number of psychiatric admissions is an important suicide risk factor in both inpatients and outpatients with schizophrenia [35,51].

Recurrent relapses, a significant severity of the disease, a descending shift in societal and occupational functioning, and a true and realistic understanding of the harmful influence of the disorder are regarded as schizophrenia-specific suicide risk factors [10]. Patients with the paranoid subtype of schizophrenia are eight times more likely to die by suicide in comparison with patients with the deficit subtype of schizophrenia [54]. Delusions are associated with more suicidal behavior in individuals with schizophrenia [53]. A research report indicates that hostility at hospital admission is linked with long-term suicidal risk [54].

Lack of adherence to antipsychotic drugs may increase suicide risk [53,55]. For example, a large follow-up study of patients released from hospitals after a hospitalization related to the first episode of schizophrenia showed that not getting antipsychotic drugs led to a 12-fold rise in the relative risk of all-cause mortality and a 37-fold rise in suicide mortality [55].

It is important to note that as a result of psychotic disorganization, an individual with schizophrenia may be involved in very unsafe, risky behavior without understanding otherwise predictable threats [29]. Such behavior may look like suicidal behavior.

5. Risk Factors Related to Comorbid Disorders

Comorbid depression and a history of suicidal behavior are important contributors to suicide risk in patients with schizophrenia [33,53,56]. One study showed that depressive symptoms, suicidal ideation and plans and a history of suicide attempts are amongst the most important forecasters of suicidal behavior in the early phases of schizophrenia [57]. Two studies suggest that patients with schizophrenia who were hospitalized after a suicide attempt had the greatest risk, of all variables examined, of dying by suicide [58,59]. Other works also indicate that suicide risk in individuals with schizophrenia is associated with mood syndromes, especially depressed mood, hopelessness and demoralization [29,33,53,60]. Panic symptoms may also contribute to suicidal behavior in patients with schizophrenia [61].

A systematic review indicates that four investigations recognized alcohol abuse as a predisposing aspect to suicidal behavior amongst individuals with schizophrenia, while three investigations recognized substance use disorders and one research investigation recognized smoking only [53]. However, one study has shown that neither alcohol nor drug abuse elevates suicide risk in individuals with schizophrenia [62]. Furthermore, a research group observed that abuse of stimulants, such as cocaine or amphetamine increases the risk of suicidal behavior in schizophrenia [63]. As noted above, the presence of medical and/or neurological disorders may increase suicide risk [16–21].

6. Risk Factors Related to Antipsychotic Medications

Some observations suggest that the side effects of antipsychotic medications may contribute to suicidality in individuals with schizophrenia [64–66]. It has been suggested that antipsychotics-induced akathisia, akinesia, tardive dyskinesia and depressogenic effects of antipsychotic medications may increase suicide risk. For example, it has been observed that there is a significant association among akathisia and suicidality in first-episode psychosis [65,66].

It is important to note that one study observed a lower suicide risk among patients with extrapyramidal symptoms [67]. The authors believe that this finding could potentially reflect greater adherence to antipsychotic treatment, exposure to higher doses, or polypharmacy in this patient group.

7. Neurobiological Aspects of Suicidal Behavior in Schizophrenia

Some lines of evidence suggest that suicidal behavior in schizophrenia has a neurobiological basis [68–73]. Dexamethasone suppression test (DST) deviations have been observed in patients with schizophrenia who attempted suicide [68,69]. For example, it has been observed that dexamethasone non-suppression may be associated with a history of suicide attempts among medication-free persons with schizophrenia [68]. Hypothalamic-pituitary-adrenal axis (HPA) hyperactivity leading to glucocorticoid neurotoxicity may be the primary way through which tissue injury occurs in several parts of the brain, as observed in neuroimaging investigations of suicide attempters with schizophrenia [70].

Some studies found lower 5-hydroxy acetic acid (5-HIAAA) levels in the cerebrospinal fluid (CSF) of suicidal patients in comparison to the CSF levels of non-suicidal individuals with schizophrenia [71,74], while other studies did not detect this difference [75–77]. One research group found that a blunted prolactin response to a D-fenfluramine administration was associated with suicidal behavior in individuals with a history of schizophrenia [78]. A significant link was found between single nucleotide polymorphisms ADRA2B rs1018351 and SLC6A3 rs403636 and a history of suicidal behavior in schizophrenia patients [73].

8. Prevention of Suicide in Patients with Schizophrenia

Suicide prevention in patients with schizophrenia is a complex task. Clinicians need to be trained in how to identify patients who are at high suicide risk. Careful management of psychotic symptoms, comorbid depression and substance use disorders is necessary to prevent suicide in individuals with schizophrenia.

Efforts in suicide prevention should focus on enhancing compliance with medications. Studies suggest that antipsychotic medications, including clozapine, risperidone, olanzapine, and quetiapine may reduce suicide risk [33,79–83].

Several studies demonstrated efficacy of clozapine for the management of suicidality in schizophrenia [81,82]. It has been proposed that this decline in suicidal behavior can be ascribed to reduction in depressive symptomatology [84]. In December 2002, the U.S. Food and Drug Administration (FDA) granted indication for clozapine to decrease the risk of recurring suicidal behavior in individuals with schizophrenia/schizoaffective disorder [50]. Potentially, early use of clozapine may significantly reduce risk of suicide in patients with schizophrenia [53]. A recent study indicates that clozapine should be administered after patients with schizophrenia fail a single antipsychotic medication trial—not until two antipsychotic drugs have been attempted, as is the existing guideline [85]. Such an approach may reduce suicidality in individuals with schizophrenia.

Other second-generation antipsychotics may also have anti-suicidal properties [33,80,86]. For example, a retrospective study of the influences of atypical antipsychotic drugs on suicidal behavior in individuals with schizophrenia or schizoaffective disorder showed that among persons who made a suicide attempt, 16.1% took second-generation antipsychotic medications, whereas in the non-suicidal group 37% took second-generation antipsychotics [80]. Another study has shown a fourfold rise in suicide attempts among individuals with schizophrenia who stopped taking olanzapine or risperidone [86].

Long-acting injections are frequently used for the treatment of psychotic disorders [87]. Observations of the effect of depot antipsychotic medications on suicide risk have produced inconsistent results. For example, Battaglia et al. [87] showed that monthly intramuscular injections of fluphenazine decanoate reduce self-harm behavior in outpatients with histories of multiple suicide attempts. Shear et al. [88] reported suicides in two young men who developed severe akathisia after treatment with depot fluphenazine. A Cochrane review by Adams and Eisenbruch [89] compared depot fluphenazine medication to oral fluphenazine for treatment of schizophrenia and found no difference between fluphenazine hydrochloride and its depot form for outcomes such as depressed mood or suicide. A meta-analysis showed that pooled long-acting antipsychotics (aripiprazole, fluphenazine, haloperidol, olanzapine, paliperidone, risperidone, and zuclopenthixol) did not differ from pooled oral antipsychotics regarding all-cause death or death due to suicide [90]. Pompilli et al. [91] suggest that long-acting injections of second-generation antipsychotics can be an effective treatment strategy to improve adherence and may result in suicide prevention by targeting modifiable suicide risk factors.

Concurrent depression is a significant risk factor for suicidal behavior in individuals with schizophrenia [29,33,34]. Studies suggest a relation between a decrease in suicide risk and the use of antidepressants [92,93]. The use of antidepressants has been associated with a decrease in all-cause mortality when used together with antipsychotic drugs [94]. Psychiatrists should consider the addition of antidepressant medications for concurrent depression in patients with schizophrenia [29,33,34]. Furthermore, medications that reduce substance abuse (e.g., naltrexone or acamprosate) should be prescribed for patients with comorbid schizophrenia/schizoaffective disorder and substance use disorder.

Non-pharmacological approaches are also important in decreasing suicidal behavior in schizophrenia [33,34,95]. Psychosocial interventions play an important role in the treatment of suicidal patients with schizophrenia. It is vital to educate mental health providers about suicidology [34]. They need to be prepared to deal with the depression, anxiety, anguish, and hopelessness of suicidal individuals with schizophrenia. Empathic care and support are critical for decreasing suicidal risk [33,34,95]. Clinicians should recognize the patient's distress, talk to the patient about his/her daily problems, and assist patients in establishing realistic goals.

Supportive, reality-orientated therapies are important in the management of patients with psychotic disorders [34]. Individual and group sessions can help patients to learn how to handle difficulties. Psychosocial interventions including cognitive-behavioral therapy, cognitive remediation, supportive therapy, supported education, training, and employment are important for successful management of schizophrenia [34,96]. One study found that cognitive therapy decreases suicidal ideation in individuals with schizophrenia [97]. Interventions such as vocational rehabilitation, social skill training, and supported employment may reduce social isolation and feeling of hopelessness, and consequently, decrease suicidality in schizophrenia patients.

Family interventions may reduce the risk of suicidal behavior, and therefore, should be a necessary component of a treatment plan of each patient with schizophrenia [98,99]. Such interventions considerably lessen rates of readmission and relapse in individuals with psychotic disorders and enhance their social and vocational performance [98,99]. Family interventions usually increase adherence to pharmacological therapy [99]. Relatives of patients with schizophrenia sometimes display excessive emotional reactions and convey intolerant, judgmental, and/or emotionally overinvolved attitudes toward patients [100–102]. Family members high in expressed emotion may cause suicidal behavior in patients with schizophrenia [100]. One of the goals of family interventions is to reduce psychological distress among family members and to decrease expressed emotion in families of patients with schizophrenia. Hence, it is essential to help families of persons with schizophrenia and to explain to patients' families that their attitude towards the patient can aid or impede recovery. It is necessary to educate families that they need to assist mental health providers to make sure that pharmacological and non-pharmacological treatments are being followed, especially after discharge from inpatient hospitalization. Families of individuals with schizophrenia need to be informed regarding manifestations of suicidality and what needs to be done if an individual with schizophrenia develops suicidal ideation, intent, or plan.

In summary, the only reliable protective factor for suicide in patients with schizophrenia is provision of and compliance with comprehensive treatment. Prevention of suicidal behavior in schizophrenia should include recognizing patients at risk, delivering the best possible therapy for psychotic symptoms, and managing comorbid depression and substance misuse. It is imperative to educate mental health and non-mental health providers about suicide prevention strategies.

Author Contributions: Conceptualization, L.S. and R.S.K.; Writing-Original Draft Preparation, L.S. and R.S.K.; Writing-Review & Editing, L.S.

Funding: This work received no external funding.

Conflicts of Interest: The authors declare no conflict of interest.

References

1. World Health Organization. Preventing Suicide. A Global Imperative. WHO, 2014. Available online: http://www.who.int/mental_health/suicide-prevention/world_report_2014/en/ (accessed on 14 January 2019).
2. Hawton, K.; van Heeringen, K. Suicide. *Lancet* **2009**, *373*, 1372–1381. [CrossRef]
3. Wyatt, R.J.; Henter, I.; Leary, M.C.; Taylor, E. An economic evaluation of schizophrenia-1991. *Soc. Psychiatry Psychiatr. Epidemiol.* **1995**, *30*, 196–205. [PubMed]

4. Jokinen, J.; Talbäck, M.; Feychting, M.; Ahlbom, A.; Ljung, R. Life expectancy after the first suicide attempt. *Acta Psychiatr. Scand.* **2018**, *137*, 287–295. [CrossRef] [PubMed]
5. Hedegaard, H.; Curtin, S.C.; Warner, M. Suicide mortality in the United States, 1999–2017. *NCHS Data Brief.* **2018**, *330*, 1–8.
6. Rutz, W.; Rihmer, Z. Suicidality in men—Practical issues, challenges, solutions. *J. Men's Health Gender* **2007**, *4*, 393–401. [CrossRef]
7. Mann, J.J. A current perspective of suicide and attempted suicide. *Ann. Intern. Med.* **2002**, *136*, 302–311. [CrossRef] [PubMed]
8. Sher, L.; Oquendo, M.A.; Mann, J.J. Risk of suicide in mood disorders. *Clin. Neurosci. Res.* **2001**, *1*, 337–344. [CrossRef]
9. Brådvik, L. Suicide risk and mental disorders. *Int. J. Environ. Res. Public Health* **2018**, *15*, 2028. [CrossRef]
10. Caldwell, C.B.; Gottesman, I.I. Schizophrenics kill themselves too: A review of risk factors for suicide. *Schizophr. Bull.* **1990**, *16*, 571–589. [CrossRef]
11. Sartorius, N.; Jablensky, A.; Korten, A.; Ernberg, G.; Anker, M.; Cooper, J.E.; Day, R. Early manifestations and first-contact incidence of schizophrenia in different cultures. A preliminary report on the initial evaluation phase of the WHO Collaborative Study on determinants of outcome of severe mental disorders. *Psychol. Med.* **1986**, *16*, 909–928. [CrossRef]
12. Sher, L. Alcohol and suicide: Neurobiological and clinical aspects. *Sci. World J.* **2006**, *21*, 700–706. [CrossRef] [PubMed]
13. Ho, R.C.; Ho, E.C.; Tai, B.C.; Ng, W.Y.; Chia, B.H. Elderly suicide with and without a history of suicidal behavior: Implications for suicide prevention and management. *Arch. Suicide Res.* **2014**, *18*, 363–375. [CrossRef]
14. Krysinska, K.; Heller, T.S.; De Leo, D. Suicide and deliberate self-harm in personality disorders. *Curr. Opin. Psychiatry* **2006**, *19*, 95–101. [CrossRef] [PubMed]
15. Choo, C.; Diederich, J.; Song, I.; Ho, R. Cluster analysis reveals risk factors for repeated suicide attempts in a multi-ethnic Asian population. *Asian J. Psychiatr.* **2014**, *8*, 38–42. [CrossRef] [PubMed]
16. Ahmedani, B.K.; Peterson, E.L.; Hu, Y.; Rossom, R.C.; Lynch, F.; Lu, C.Y.; Waitzfelder, B.E.; Owen-Smith, A.A.; Hubley, S.; Prabhakar, D.; et al. Major physical health conditions and risk of suicide. *Am. J. Prev. Med.* **2017**, *53*, 308–315. [CrossRef]
17. Elman, I.; Borsook, D.; Volkow, N.D. Pain and suicidality: Insights from reward and addiction neuroscience. *Prog. Neurobiol.* **2013**, *109*, 1–27. [CrossRef] [PubMed]
18. Rogers, M.L.; Joiner, T.E. Interactive effects of acute suicidal affective disturbance and pain persistence on suicide attempt frequency and lethality. *Crisis* **2019**, in press. [CrossRef]
19. King, S.A. Opioids, Suicide, Mental Disorders, and Pain. *Psychiatr. Times* **2018**, *35*, 11. Available online: https://www.psychiatrictimes.com/psychopharmacology/opioids-suicide-mental-disorders-and-pain (accessed on 24 April 2019).
20. Coughlin, S.S.; Sher, L. Suicidal behavior and neurological illnesses. *J. Depress. Anxiety* **2013**, *9*, 12443.
21. Oquendo, M.A.; Friedman, J.H.; Grunebaum, M.F.; Burke, A.; Silver, J.M.; Mann, J.J. Suicidal behavior and mild traumatic brain injury in major depression. *J. Nerv. Ment. Dis.* **2004**, *192*, 430–434. [CrossRef]
22. Brent, D. Prevention programs to augment family and child resilience can have lasting effects on suicidal risk. *Suicide Life Threat. Behav.* **2016**, *46*, S39–S47. [CrossRef] [PubMed]
23. Sher, L. Is it possible to predict suicide? *Aust. N. Z. J. Psychiatry* **2011**, *45*, 341. [CrossRef]
24. Varese, F.; Smeets, F.; Drukker, M.; Lieverse, R.; Lataster, T.; Viechtbauer, W.; Read, J.; van Os, J.; Bentall, R.P. Childhood adversities increase the risk of psychosis: A meta-analysis of patient-control, prospective-and cross-sectional cohort studies. *Schizophr. Bull.* **2012**, *38*, 661–671. [CrossRef] [PubMed]
25. Serafini, G.; Muzio, C.; Piccinini, G.; Flouri, E.; Ferrigno, G.; Pompili, M.; Girardi, P.; Amore, M. Life adversities and suicidal behavior in young individuals: A systematic review. *Eur. Child. Adolesc. Psychiatry* **2015**, *24*, 1423–1446. [CrossRef] [PubMed]
26. Bleuler, E. *Dementia Praecox: oder Gruppe der Schizophrenien*; Franz Deuticke: Leipzig, Germany, 1911.
27. Kraepelin, E. Psychiatrische Randbemerkungen zur Zeitgeschichte. *Suddeutsch. Monatshefte* **1919**, *2*, 171–183. [CrossRef]
28. Rennie, T.A.C. Follow-up study of five hundred patients with schizophrenia admitted to the hospital from 1913 to 1923. *Arch. Neurol. Psychiatry* **1939**, *42*, 877–891. [CrossRef]

29. Siris, S.G. Suicide and schizophrenia. *J. Psychopharmacol.* **2001**, *15*, 127–135. [CrossRef] [PubMed]
30. Cohen, S.; Lavelle, J.; Rich, C.L.; Bromet, E. Rates and correlates of suicide attempts in first-admission psychotic patients. *Acta Psychiatr. Scand.* **1994**, *90*, 167–171. [CrossRef]
31. Gupta, S.; Black, D.W.; Arndt, S.; Hubbard, W.C.; Andreasen, N.C. Factors associated with suicide attempts among patients with schizophrenia. *Psychiatr. Serv.* **1998**, *49*, 1353–1355. [CrossRef]
32. White, J.; Gray, R.; Jones, M. The development of the serious mental illness physical Health Improvement Profile. *J. Psychiatr. Ment. Health Nurs.* **2009**, *16*, 493–498. [CrossRef]
33. Balhara, Y.P.; Verma, R. Schizophrenia and suicide. *East. Asian Arch. Psychiatry* **2012**, *22*, 126–133. [PubMed]
34. Roy, A.; Pompili, M. Management of schizophrenia with suicide risk. *Psychiatr. Clin. N. Am.* **2009**, *32*, 863–883. [CrossRef] [PubMed]
35. Popovic, D.; Benabarre, A.; Crespo, J.M.; Goikolea, J.M.; González-Pinto, A.; Gutiérrez-Rojas, L.; Montes, J.M.; Vieta, E. Risk factors for suicide in schizophrenia: Systematic review and clinical recommendations. *Acta Psychiatr. Scand.* **2014**, *130*, 418–426. [CrossRef] [PubMed]
36. Verma, D.; Srivastava, M.K.; Singh, S.K.; Bhatia, T.; Deshpande, S.N. Lifetime suicide intent, executive function and insight in schizophrenia and schizoaffective disorders. *Schizophr. Res.* **2016**, *178*, 12–16. [CrossRef] [PubMed]
37. Black, D.W.; Winokur, G.; Warrack, G. Suicide in schizophrenia: The Iowa Record Linkage Study. *J. Clin. Psychiatry* **1985**, *46*, 14–17. [PubMed]
38. Copas, J.B.; Robin, A. Suicide in psychiatric in-patients. *Br. J. Psychiatry* **1982**, *141*, 503–511. [CrossRef] [PubMed]
39. Newman, S.C.; Bland, R.C. Mortality in a cohort of patients with schizophrenia: A record linkage study. *Can. J. Psychiatry* **1991**, *36*, 239–245. [CrossRef] [PubMed]
40. Breier, A.; Astrachan, B.M. Characterization of schizophrenic patients who commit suicide. *Am. J. Psychiatry* **1984**, *141*, 206–209.
41. Roy, A. Suicide in chronic schizophrenia. *Br. J. Psychiatry* **1982**, *141*, 171–177. [CrossRef]
42. Harkavy-Friedman, J.M.; Nelson, E. Management of the suicidal patient with schizophrenia. *Psychiatr. Clin. North. Am.* **1997**, *20*, 625–640. [CrossRef]
43. Inamdar, S.C.; Lewis, D.O.; Siomopoulos, G.; Shanok, S.S.; Lamela, M. Violent and suicidal behavior in psychotic adolescents. *Am. J. Psychiatry* **1982**, *139*, 932–935. [PubMed]
44. Roy, A.; Mazonson, A.; Pickar, D. Attempted suicide in chronic schizophrenia. *Br. J. Psychiatry* **1984**, *144*, 303–306. [CrossRef] [PubMed]
45. Niskanen, P. Treatment results achieved in psychiatric day hospital care: A follow-up of 100 patients. *Acta Psychiatr. Scand.* **1974**, *50*, 401–409. [CrossRef] [PubMed]
46. Nordentoft, M.; Madsen, T.; Fedyszyn, I. Suicidal behavior and mortality in first-episode psychosis. *J. Nerv. Ment. Dis.* **2015**, *203*, 387–392. [CrossRef] [PubMed]
47. Tsuang, M.T.; Woolson, R.F. Excess mortality in schizophrenia and affective disorders. Do suicides and accidental deaths solely account for this excess? *Arch. Gen. Psychiatry* **1978**, *35*, 1181–1185. [CrossRef] [PubMed]
48. Barrett, E.A.; Sundet, K.; Faerden, A.; Nesvåg, R.; Agartz, I.; Fosse, R.; Mork, E.; Steen, N.E.; Andreassen, O.A.; Melle, I. Suicidality before and in the early phases of first episode psychosis. *Schizophr. Res.* **2010**, *119*, 11–17. [CrossRef]
49. Chan, S.K.W.; Chan, S.W.Y.; Pang, H.H.; Yan, K.K.; Hui, C.L.M.; Chang, W.C.; Lee, E.H.M.; Chen, E.Y.H. Association of an early intervention service for psychosis with suicide rate among patients with first-episode schizophrenia-spectrum disorders. *JAMA Psychiatry* **2018**, *75*, 458–464. [CrossRef]
50. Ventriglio, A.; Gentile, A.; Bonfitto, I.; Stella, E.; Mari, M.; Steardo, L.; Bellomo, A. Suicide in the early stage of schizophrenia. *Front. Psychiatry* **2016**, *7*, 116. [CrossRef]
51. Carlborg, A.; Winnerbäck, K.; Jönsson, E.G.; Jokinen, J.; Nordström, P. Suicide in schizophrenia. *Expert Rev. Neurother.* **2010**, *10*, 1153–1164. [CrossRef]
52. Hawton, K.; Sutton, L.; Haw, C.; Sinclair, J.; Deeks, J.J. Schizophrenia and suicide: Systematic review of risk factors. *Br. J. Psychiatry* **2005**, *187*, 9–20. [CrossRef]
53. Hor, K.; Taylor, M. Suicide and schizophrenia: A systematic review of rates and risk factors. *J. Psychopharmacol.* **2010**, *24*, 81–90. [CrossRef]

54. Fenton, W.S.; McGlashan, T.H.; Victor, B.J.; Blyler, C.R. Symptoms, subtype, and suicidality in patients with schizophrenia spectrum disorders. *Am. J. Psychiatry* **1997**, *154*, 199–204. [PubMed]
55. Tiihonen, J.; Wahlbeck, K.; Lönnqvist, J.; Klaukka, T.; Ioannidis, J.P.; Volavka, J.; Haukka, J. Effectiveness of antipsychotic treatments in a nationwide cohort of patients in community care after first hospitalisation due to schizophrenia and schizoaffective disorder: Observational follow-up study. *BMJ* **2006**, *333*, 224. [CrossRef] [PubMed]
56. Hettige, N.C.; Bani-Fatemi, A.; Sakinofsky, I.; De Luca, V. A biopsychosocial evaluation of the risk for suicide in schizophrenia. *CNS Spectr.* **2018**, *23*, 253–263. [CrossRef] [PubMed]
57. Bertelsen, M.; Jeppesen, P.; Petersen, L.; Thorup, A.; Øhlenschlaeger, J.; le Quach, P.; Christensen, T.Ø.; Krarup, G.; Jørgensen, P.; Nordentoft, M. Suicidal behaviour and mortality in first-episode psychosis: The OPUS trial. *Br. J. Psychiatry* **2007**, *51*, s140–s146. [CrossRef]
58. Reutfors, J.; Brandt, L.; Jönsson, E.G.; Ekbom, A.; Sparén, P.; Osby, U. Risk factors for suicide in schizophrenia: Findings from a Swedish population-based case-control study. *Schizophr. Res.* **2009**, *108*, 231–237. [CrossRef] [PubMed]
59. Sinclair, J.M.; Mullee, M.A.; King, E.A.; Baldwin, DS. Suicide in schizophrenia: A retrospective case-control study of 51 suicides. *Schizophr. Bull.* **2004**, *30*, 803–811. [CrossRef]
60. Saarinen, P.I.; Lehtonen, J.; Lönnqvist, J. Suicide risk in schizophrenia: An analysis of 17 consecutive suicides. *Schizophr. Bull.* **1999**, *25*, 533–542. [CrossRef]
61. Goodwin, R.; Lyons, J.S.; McNally, R.J. Panic attacks in schizophrenia. *Schizophr. Res.* **2002**, *58*, 213–220. [CrossRef]
62. McGirr, A.; Turecki, G. What is specific to suicide in schizophrenia disorder? Demographic, clinical and behavioural dimensions. *Schizophr. Res.* **2008**, *98*, 217–224. [CrossRef]
63. González-Pinto, A.; Aldama, A.; González, C.; Mosquera, F.; Arrasate, M.; Vieta, E. Predictors of suicide in first-episode affective and nonaffective psychotic inpatients: Five-year follow-up of patients from a catchment area in Vitoria, Spain. *J. Clin. Psychiatry* **2007**, *68*, 242–247. [CrossRef] [PubMed]
64. Aguilar, E.J.; Siris, S.G. Do antipsychotic drugs influence suicidal behavior in schizophrenia? *Psychopharmacol. Bull.* **2007**, *40*, 128–142. [PubMed]
65. Seemüller, F.; Schennach, R.; Mayr, A.; Musil, R.; Jäger, M.; Maier, W.; Klingenberg, S.; Heuser, I.; Klosterkötter, J.; Gastpar, M.; et al. German Study Group on First-Episode Schizophrenia. Akathisia and suicidal ideation in first-episode schizophrenia. *J. Clin. Psychopharmacol.* **2012**, *32*, 694–698. [CrossRef] [PubMed]
66. Seemüller, F.; Lewitzka, U.; Bauer, M.; Meyer, S.; Musil, R.; Schennach, R.; Riedel, M.; Doucette, S.; Möller, H.J. The relationship of Akathisia with treatment emergent suicidality among patients with first-episode schizophrenia treated with haloperidol or risperidone. *Pharmacopsychiatry* **2012**, *45*, 292–296. [CrossRef] [PubMed]
67. Reutfors, J.; Clapham, E.; Bahmanyar, S.; Brandt, L.; Jönsson, E.G.; Ekbom, A.; Bodén, R.; Ösby, U. Suicide risk and antipsychotic side effects in schizophrenia: Nested case-control study. *Hum. Psychopharmacol.* **2016**, *31*, 341–345. [CrossRef] [PubMed]
68. Jones, J.S.; Stein, D.J.; Stanley, B.; Guido, J.R.; Winchel, R.; Stanley, M. Negative and depressive symptoms in suicidal schizophrenics. *Acta Psychiatr. Scand.* **1994**, *89*, 81–87. [CrossRef]
69. Płocka-Lewandowska, M.; Araszkiewicz, A.; Rybakowski, J.K. Dexamethasone suppression test and suicide attempts in schizophrenic patients. *Eur. Psychiatry* **2001**, *16*, 428–431. [CrossRef]
70. Bradley, A.J.; Dinan, T.G. A systematic review of hypothalamic-pituitary-adrenal axis function in schizophrenia: Implications for mortality. *J. Psychopharmacol.* **2010**, *24*, 91–118. [CrossRef]
71. Cooper, S.J.; Kelly, C.B.; King, D.J. 5-Hydroxyindoleacetic acid in cerebrospinal fluid and prediction of suicidal behaviour in schizophrenia. *Lancet* **1992**, *340*, 940–941. [CrossRef]
72. Kim, S.; Choi, K.H.; Baykiz, A.F.; Gershenfeld, H.K. Suicide candidate genes associated with bipolar disorder and schizophrenia: An exploratory gene expression profiling analysis of post-mortem prefrontal cortex. *BMC Genom.* **2007**, *8*, 413. [CrossRef]
73. Molnar, S.; Mihanović, M.; Grah, M.; Kezić, S.; Filaković, P.; Degmecić, D. Comparative study on gene tags of the neurotransmission system in schizophrenic and suicidal subjects. *Coll. Antropol.* **2010**, *34*, 1427–1432. [PubMed]

74. Neider, D.; Lindström, L.H.; Bodén, R. Risk factors for suicide among patients with schizophrenia: A cohort study focused on cerebrospinal fluid levels of homovanillic acid and 5-hydroxyindoleacetic acid. *Neuropsychiatr. Dis. Treat.* **2016**, *12*, 1711–1714. [CrossRef] [PubMed]
75. Roy, A.; Ninan, P.; Mazonson, A.; Pickar, D.; Van Kammen, D.; Linnoila, M.; Paul, S.M. CSF monoamine metabolites in chronic schizophrenic patients who attempt suicide. *Psychol. Med.* **1985**, *15*, 335–340. [CrossRef] [PubMed]
76. Lemus, C.Z.; Lieberman, J.A.; Johns, C.A.; Pollack, S.; Bookstein, P.; Cooper, T.B. CSF 5-hydroxyindoleacetic acid levels and suicide attempts in schizophrenia. *Biol. Psychiatry* **1990**, *27*, 926–929. [CrossRef]
77. Carlborg, A.; Jokinen, J.; Nordström, A.L.; Jönsson, E.G.; Nordström, P. CSF 5-HIAA, attempted suicide and suicide risk in schizophrenia spectrum psychosis. *Schizophr. Res.* **2009**, *112*, 80–85. [CrossRef]
78. Corrêa, H.; Duval, F.; Mokrani, M.C.; Bailey, P.; Trémeau, F.; Staner, L.; Diep, T.S.; Crocq, M.A.; Macher, J.P. Serotonergic function and suicidal behavior in schizophrenia. *Schizophr. Res.* **2002**, *56*, 75–85. [CrossRef]
79. Keck, P.E., Jr.; Strakowski, S.M.; McElroy, S.L. The efficacy of atypical antipsychotics in the treatment of depressive symptoms, hostility, and suicidality in patients with schizophrenia. *J. Clin. Psychiatry* **2000**, *61*, 4–9.
80. Barak, Y.; Mirecki, I.; Knobler, H.Y.; Natan, Z.; Aizenberg, D. Suicidality and second generation antipsychotics in schizophrenia patients: A case-controlled retrospective study during a 5-year period. *Psychopharmacology* **2004**, *175*, 215–219. [CrossRef]
81. Meltzer, H.Y.; Alphs, L.; Green, A.I.; Altamura, A.C.; Anand, R.; Bertoldi, A.; Bourgeois, M.; Chouinard, G.; Islam, M.Z.; Kane, J.; et al. International Suicide Prevention Trial Study Group. Clozapine treatment for suicidality in schizophrenia: International Suicide Prevention Trial (InterSePT). *Arch. Gen. Psychiatry* **2003**, *60*, 82–91. [CrossRef]
82. Sernyak, M.J.; Desai, R.; Stolar, M.; Rosenheck, R. Impact of clozapine on completed suicide. *Am. J. Psychiatry* **2001**, *158*, 931–937. [CrossRef]
83. Tiihonen, J.; Mittendorfer-Rutz, E.; Majak, M.; Mehtälä, J.; Hoti, F.; Jedenius, E.; Enkusson, D.; Leval, A.; Sermon, J.; Tanskanen, A.; et al. Real-world effectiveness of antipsychotic treatments in a Nationwide Cohort of 29,823 patients with schizophrenia. *JAMA Psychiatry* **2017**, *74*, 686–693. [CrossRef] [PubMed]
84. Saunders, K.E.; Hawton, K. The role of psychopharmacology in suicide prevention. *Epidemiol. Psichiatr. Soc.* **2009**, *18*, 172–178. [CrossRef] [PubMed]
85. Kahn, R.S.; Winter van Rossum, I.; Leucht, S.; McGuire, P.; Lewis, S.W.; Leboyer, M.; Arango, C.; Dazzan, P.; Drake, R.; Heres, S.; et al. Amisulpride and olanzapine followed by open-label treatment with clozapine in first-episode schizophrenia and schizophreniform disorder (OPTiMiSE): A three-phase switching study. *Lancet Psychiatry* **2018**, *5*, 797–807. [CrossRef]
86. Herings, R.M.; Erkens, J.A. Increased suicide attempt rate among patients interrupting use of atypical antipsychotics. *Pharmacoepidemiol. Drug Saf.* **2003**, *12*, 423–424. [CrossRef] [PubMed]
87. Battaglia, J.; Wolff, T.K.; Wagner-Johnson, D.S.; Rush, A.J.; Carmody, T.J.; Basco, M.R. Structured diagnostic assessment and depot fluphenazine treatment of multiple suicide attempters in the emergency department. *Int. Clin. Psychopharmacol.* **1999**, *14*, 361–372. [CrossRef] [PubMed]
88. Shear, M.K.; Frances, A.; Weiden, P. Suicide associated with akathisia and depot fluphenazine treatment. *J. Clin. Psychopharmacol.* **1983**, *3*, 235–236. [CrossRef]
89. Adams, C.E.; Eisenbruch, M. Depot fluphenazine for schizophrenia. *Cochrane Database Syst. Rev.* **2000**, *2*, CD000307.
90. Kishi, T.; Matsunaga, S.; Iwata, N. Mortality risk associated with long-acting injectable antipsychotics: A systematic review and meta-analyses of randomized controlled trials. *Schizophr. Bull.* **2016**, *42*, 1438–1445. [CrossRef]
91. Pompili, M.; Orsolini, L.; Lamis, D.A.; Goldsmith, D.R.; Nardella, A.; Falcone, G.; Corigliano, V.; Luciano, M.; Fiorillo, A. Suicide prevention in schizophrenia: Do long-acting injectable antipsychotics (LAIs) have a role? *CNS Neurol. Disord. Drug Targets* **2017**, *16*, 454–462. [CrossRef]
92. Henriksson, S.; Isacsson, G. Increased antidepressant use and fewer suicides in Jämtland county, Sweden, after a primary care educational programme on the treatment of depression. *Acta Psychiatr. Scand.* **2006**, *114*, 159–167. [CrossRef]
93. Isacsson, G.; Rich, C.L. Antidepressant drug use and suicide prevention. *Int. Rev. Psychiatry* **2005**, *17*, 153–162. [CrossRef] [PubMed]

94. Haukka, J.; Tiihonen, J.; Härkänen, T.; Lönnqvist, J. Association between medication and risk of suicide, attempted suicide and death in nationwide cohort of suicidal patients with schizophrenia. *Pharmacoepidemiol. Drug Saf.* **2008**, *17*, 686–696. [CrossRef] [PubMed]
95. Cotton, P.G.; Drake, R.E.; Gates, C. Critical treatment issues in suicide among schizophrenics. *Hosp. Community Psychiatry* **1985**, *36*, 534–536. [CrossRef] [PubMed]
96. Kahn, R.S.; Sommer, I.E.; Murray, R.M.; Meyer-Lindenberg, A.; Weinberger, D.R.; Cannon, T.D.; O'Donovan, M.; Correll, C.U.; Kane, J.M.; van Os, J.; et al. Schizophrenia. *Nat. Rev. Dis. Primers* **2015**, *1*, 15067. [CrossRef] [PubMed]
97. Bateman, K.; Hansen, L.; Turkington, D.; Kingdon, D. Cognitive behavioral therapy reduces suicidal ideation in schizophrenia: Results from a randomized controlled trial. *Suicide Life Threat. Behav.* **2007**, *37*, 284–290. [CrossRef] [PubMed]
98. McFarlane, W.R.; Dixon, L.; Lukens, E.; Lucksted, A. Family psychoeducation and schizophrenia: A review of the literature. *J. Marital Fam. Ther.* **2003**, *29*, 223–245. [CrossRef] [PubMed]
99. Onwumere, J.; Bebbington, P.; Kuipers, E. Family interventions in early psychosis: Specificity and effectiveness. *Epidemiol. Psychiatr. Sci.* **2011**, *20*, 113–119. [CrossRef]
100. Demir, S. The relationship between expressed emotion and the probability of suicide among Turkish psychiatric outpatients: A descriptive cross-sectional survey. *Fam. Community Health* **2018**, *41*, 111–116. [CrossRef]
101. Napa, W.; Tungpunkom, P.; Pothimas, N. Effectiveness of family interventions on psychological distress and expressed emotion in family members of individuals diagnosed with first-episode psychosis: A systematic review. *JBI Database Syst. Rev. Implement. Rep.* **2017**, *15*, 1057–1079. [CrossRef]
102. Amaresha, A.C.; Venkatasubramanian, G. Expressed emotion in schizophrenia: An overview. *Indian J. Psychol. Med.* **2012**, *34*, 12–20.

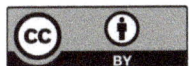

© 2019 by the authors. Licensee MDPI, Basel, Switzerland. This article is an open access article distributed under the terms and conditions of the Creative Commons Attribution (CC BY) license (http://creativecommons.org/licenses/by/4.0/).

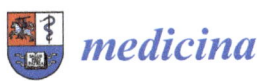

Review
Suicidality in Borderline Personality Disorder

Joel Paris *

Institute of Community and Family Psychiatry, McGill University, 4333 chemin de la cote ste. Catherine, Montreal, QC H3T1E4, Canada

Received: 9 January 2019; Accepted: 15 May 2019; Published: 28 May 2019

Abstract: Borderline personality disorder (BPD) is associated with suicidal behaviors and self-harm. Up to 10% of BPD patients will die by suicide. However, no research data support the effectiveness of suicide prevention in this disorder, and hospitalization has not been shown to be useful. The most evidence-based treatment methods for BPD are specifically designed psychotherapies.

Keywords: suicide suicidality personality disorder; borderline personality disorder; self-harm

1. Introduction

This review is based on a search with the key words "borderline personality disorder" and "suicide or suicidality" in MEDLINE and PsycINFO of all articles since 2000 (along with some important older articles). This review focuses on articles that are most relevant to the following questions:

(1) What suicidal behaviors are seen in patients with borderline personality disorder (BPD), and what is their motivation?
(2) What is the risk for death by suicide in BPD?
(3) Is there evidence for the value of hospitalizing suicidal BPD patients?
(4) What are the most evidence-based treatments for suicidal BPD patients?

2. Suicidal Behaviors in BPD

As defined by the DSM-5 [1] and by the ICD-11 [2], personality disorders (PDs) are characterized by abnormal patterns of inner experience and behavior. These affect cognition, emotion, interpersonal functioning, impulse control, are inflexible and pervasive, lead to clinically significant distress or impairment, are stable and of long duration, and have an onset in adolescence or early adulthood. Personality disorders are common in practice, and can be found, above and beyond other diagnoses, in up to 45% of all outpatients [3]. Of these, BPD is by far the most researched category due to the clinical challenges it presents.

BPD is associated with a wide range of psychopathology, including unstable mood, impulsive behaviors, as well as unstable interpersonal relationships [1]. BPD patients have a mean of three lifetime suicide attempts, mostly by overdose [4].

Self-harm behaviors (i.e., non-suicidal self-injury) (NSSI) [5], are also common in BPD. NSSI usually presents as superficial cuts to the wrists and arms. However, NSSI is not suicidal in intent; BPD patients have problems with emotional regulation and cut themselves addictively to reduce painful inner states [6]. Cutting relieves emotional tension, but does not reflect a wish to die [7].

While drug overdoses can sometimes be life threatening, these behaviors vary greatly in nature and intent. They usually occur following stressful life events, and patients describe their motivation as a wish to escape [7]. Most incidents reflect ambivalent motivation, involving small quantities of medication and/or calling significant others for help. Even when potentially fatal overdoses occur, patients often contact people who are in a position to intervene.

It has long been established that suicide attempters and completers are separate but overlapping populations [8]. In a large-scale follow-up of attempters seen in an emergency room (ER), only about

3% eventually died by suicide [9]. Most repetitive attempts occur in young women, and decrease with time [10].

3. Death by Suicide in BPD Patients

Follow-back research has found that suicide occurs in up to 10% of BPD cases [11,12]. However, lower rates (3%–6%) have been reported in prospectively followed cohorts [13–15]. These discrepancies could reflect less-severe suicidality in patients who agree to be followed in research studies.

By and large, suicides in BPD occur later in the course of the illness and follow long courses of unsuccessful treatment [16]. A 15-year follow-back study found that the mean age at suicide to be 30 [12], while a 27-year follow-up reported a mean age of 37, with a standard deviation of 10 [11]. Thus, patients are not at their highest risk of suicide when they are young and frequent visitors to the ER.

Even so, patients with BPD do kill themselves. Psychological autopsy methods, which involve post-mortem interviews with families, have examined the frequency of this diagnosis in death by suicide [17–19]. In these studies, PDs were present in about half of the cases under the age of 35, with BPD being the most common category.

A meta-analysis by Pompili et al. [20] noted that suicidality is "more alarming" in young people, with a high level of suicidal behaviors. Yet the great majority of BPD patients eventually improve over time [16], and those who die by suicide tend to be those who fail to recover.

Males with BPD have a different pattern. Nearly a third of youth suicides, most of whom are male, can be diagnosed with BPD by psychological autopsy [17]. Other studies of BPD patients who died by suicide also show a preponderance of males [21]. Few of these patients were in treatment at the time of their death.

4. Hospitalization for Suicidality in BPD Patients

Many BPD patients have courses of treatment marked by multiple failed suicide attempts. These treatments are associated with multiple trials of psychotherapy, multiple prescriptions, repeated emergency room visits, and hospitalization for suicide attempts and threats [22]. Yet the research literature on the management of suicidality in BPD does not provide evidence-based guidelines for the prevention of death by suicide [23].

It has long been known that clinicians lack algorithms that can predict a fatal outcome in major mental disorders with any accuracy. As summarized in an article in The Lancet [24], in spite of a large body of research on suicide prediction, there is still no effective algorithm that can be used in practice to predict suicide. At best, clinicians are left with guidelines that may be commonsensical, but that lack empirical support.

However, the absence of evidence for prevention has not changed practice in managing BPD. Specifically, many patients are admitted to hospital when they attempt or threaten suicide. It is understandable that clinicians want to err on the safe side, but the absence of controlled data prevents us from concluding that hospital stays offer an effective method of suicide prevention. Admission for suicidal threats was recommended by the American Psychiatric Association guidelines for the treatment of BPD [25]. However, these guidelines, which have never been updated, were based on clinical opinion, and not on data showing that hospital admission has a preventive effect.

Repeated hospitalization for suicidal threats and attempts can also be counter-productive, since it interferes with out-patient treatment, and makes it impossible for patients to remain in the workplace [26–28]. It can also lead to a kind of "regression", with an increase of symptoms based on the behavioral reinforcement of suicidal behavior. Linehan [6] recommends not admitting patients for suicidality beyond an overnight hold in a crisis.

5. Evidence-Based Treatments for BPD

We now know that well-structured ambulatory treatment, using methods specifically developed for BPD, is an effective intervention for most BPD patients. The most extensively investigated treatment is dialectical behavior therapy (DBT) [6], whose efficacy has been confirmed by randomized clinical trials [29,30]. The main outcomes are reductions in overdoses, in emergency room visits for suicidality, reduced frequency of self-harm, and reduced hospital admissions. DBT specifically aims to modify the regulation of emotion, teaching patients how to regulate negative emotions in ways other than cutting or overdosing [6].

Several other psychotherapy methods have also been tested in randomized clinical trials: mentalization-based therapy [31,32]; transference-focused psychotherapy [33]; schema-focused therapy [34]; and standard cognitive therapy [35].

All these methods target the affective instability (emotion dysregulation) that characterizes BPD [6,36], as well as impulsivity [37]. Emotion dysregulation accompanied by a lack of control over impulses makes patients more likely to turn to suicidal actions, and the frequency of suicide attempts is strongly related to these traits [10]. Thus, all methods of psychotherapy attempt to teach patients to stand outside their emotions, to self-reflect before acting on them, and to develop a better understanding of interpersonal conflict.

By and large, all psychological treatments that are well-structured and specifically designed for BPD patients are superior to standard clinical management. A Cochrane report [38] as well as a systematic meta-analysis [39] have summarized this evidence, supporting the conclusion that specific forms of psychotherapy for BPD are efficacious. These methods are usually provided in out-patient settings, and do not require hospital admission. As noted by Zanarini [40], BPD patients need to "get a life", which means therapists must work actively to involve them with life goals, such as career and social networks.

In contrast, the efficacy of pharmacological agents in BPD is not well established. No clinical trials have documented remission of the disorder with successful drug treatment, and a Cochrane report did not find sufficient evidence to prescribe *any* drug for patients with BPD [41]. Recent research has also shown that anticonvulsant mood stabilizers are not efficacious [42]. There is some evidence for the use of antipsychotics for short periods [43]. A similar conclusion has been reached by the UK National Institute on Clinical Excellence [44]. Unfortunately, it has long been observed that most BPD patients are often on multiple medications, including antidepressants, mood stabilizers, and/or neuroleptics [22], and this practice does not seem to have changed. These interventions do not require hospital admission. There is also no evidence that pharmacological regimes are effective for suicide prevention.

6. Implications for Practice

One of the most unique aspects of BPD is chronic suicidal ideation [27]. Patients with mood disorders can be suicidal when depressed, but usually put these ideas aside when they go into remission. In contrast, BPD patients may consider suicide on a daily basis for months to years, and only go into remission much later. Suicidal ideas will vary in intensity over time, waxing when life events are stressful, and waning when they are not.

Yet by themselves, suicidal thoughts are too common to be useful in predicting suicidal actions. But while patients with suicidal behaviors have a statistically higher risk, one cannot predict who is most likely to die by suicide. Deaths by suicide are rare events relative to attempts, which is why large-scale follow-up studies have found that algorithms based on risk factors fail to predict who will die by suicide [45,46]. The problem is false positives (patients who fit a profile but never kill themselves).

Most patients with BPD, despite having suicidal thoughts for long periods of time and multiple suicide attempts, never kill themselves. Thus, the level of alarm created by patients with BPD who present in clinics and ERs with suicidal ideas is not necessarily justified, even when threats are dramatic or blood-curdling. Clinicians need to work on making these patents more functional, and should not be distracted from these therapeutic tasks by suicidality.

Needless to say, chronic suicidality can be draining for therapists, and no one wants to lose a patient in this way. Yet in BPD, suicidality "goes with the territory" [47], and most patients cannot be treated without accepting a calculated risk [48]. Moreover, recommending ER visits and hospitalization reinforces the very behaviors they are designed to treat [6].

Hospitalization has not been supported by evidence, and when suicidality is chronic, admission to hospital provides only temporary relief; most patients continue to have suicidal ideas after discharge. While some research describes intensive treatment in hospital [49], similar programs could be offered on an out-patient basis. To avoid the harm of repetitive admissions, one might prefer day treatment, which offers the advantages of admission (intensive treatment by an experienced team) without its disadvantages, and has some supporting evidence for its efficacy [31]. Unfortunately, day programs usually have waiting lists and are not useful in a crisis.

In practice, BPD patients are commonly held in ERs (or admitted to wards) when they threaten suicide, cut themselves, or overdose. These choices are partly determined by a fear of litigation. However, to minimize the risk of lawsuits, clinicians can ensure careful record keeping, consult frequently with colleagues, and get families involved early on in treatment [50].

Based on current evidence, it is reasonable to conclude that we should treat suicidal patients with BPD on an out-patient basis using specialized forms of psychotherapy. Psychopharmacology remains adjunctive and optional. Hospital admission can be justified by either a near-fatal attempt (requiring a re-evaluation), or a micro-psychotic episode (requiring pharmacological intervention) [27]. Since we have no firm evidence that death by suicide in BPD can be prevented, we should focus on providing existing evidence-based psychological treatments designed for this challenging population.

Funding: This research received no external funding.

Conflicts of Interest: The authors declare no conflicts of interest.

References

1. American Psychiatric Association. *Diagnostic and Statistical Manual of Mental Disorders*, 5th ed.; Text Revision; American Psychiatric Press: Washington DC, USA, 2013.
2. World Health Organization. *International Classification of Diseases*, 11th ed.; World Health Organization: Geneva, Switzerland, 2018.
3. Zimmerman, M.; Rothschild, L.; Chelminski, I. The prevalence of DSM-IV personality disorders in psychiatric outpatients. *Am. J. Psychiatry* **2005**, *162*, 1911–1918. [CrossRef]
4. Soloff, P.H.; Lynch, K.G.; Kelly, T.M.; Malone, K.M.; Mann, J.J. Characteristics of suicide attempts of patients with major depressive episode and borderline personality disorder: A comparative study. *Am. J. Psychiatry* **2000**, *157*, 601–608. [CrossRef] [PubMed]
5. Nock, M.K.; Favazza, A. Nonsuicidal self-injury: Definition and classification. In *Understanding Nonsuicidal Self- Injury: Origins, Assessment, and Treatment*; Nock, M.K., Ed.; American Psychological Association: Washington, DC, USA, 2009; pp. 9–18.
6. Linehan, M.M. *Cognitive Behavioral Therapy of Borderline Personality Disorder*; Guilford: New York, NY, USA, 1993.
7. Brown, M.Z.; Comtois, K.A.; Linehan, M.M. Reasons for suicide attempts and nonsuicidal self-injury in women with borderline personality disorder. *J. Abnorm. Psychol.* **2002**, *111*, 198–202. [CrossRef]
8. Beautrais, A.L. Suicides and serious suicide attempts: Two populations or one? *Psychol. Med.* **2001**, *31*, 837–845. [CrossRef] [PubMed]
9. Hawton, K.; Zahl, D.; Weatherall, R. Suicide following deliberate self-harm: Long-term follow-up of patients who presented to a general hospital. *Br. J. Psychiatry* **2003**, *182*, 537–542. [CrossRef] [PubMed]
10. Paris, J. *The Treatment of Borderline Personality Disorder*, 2nd ed.; Guilford: New York, NY, USA, 2019.
11. Paris, J.; Zweig-Frank, H. A twenty-seven year follow-up of borderline patients. *Compr. Psychiatry* **2001**, *42*, 482–487. [CrossRef]
12. Stone, M.H. *The Fate of Borderline Patients*; Guilford: New York, NY, USA, 1990.

13. Gunderson, J.G.; Stout, R.L.; McGlashan, T.H.; Shea, T.; Morey, L.C.; Grilo, C.M.; Zanarini, M.C.; Yen, S.; Markowitz, J.C.; Sanislow, C.; et al. Ten-year course of Borderline Personality Disorder: Psychopathology and function from the Collaborative Longitudinal Personality Disorders Study. *Arch. Gen. Psychiatry* **2011**, *68*, 827–837. [CrossRef] [PubMed]
14. Zanarini, M.C.; Frankenburg, F.; Reich, B.; Fitzmaurice, G. Attainment and stability of sustained symptomatic remission and recovery among borderline patients and Axis II comparison subjects: A 16-year prospective followup study. *Am. J. Psychiatry* **2012**, *169*, 476–483. [CrossRef]
15. Temes, C.M.; Frankenburg, F.; Fitzmaurice, G.; Zanarini, M.C. Deaths by suicide and other causes among patients with borderline personality disorder and personality-disordered comparison subjects over 24 years of prospective follow-up. *J. Clin. Psychiatry* **2019**, in press. [CrossRef]
16. Paris, J. *Personality Disorders Over Time*; American Psychiatric Press: Washington, DC, USA, 2003.
17. Lesage, A.D.; Boyer, R.; Grunberg, F.; Morisette, R.; Vanier, C.; Morrisette, R.; Ménard-Buteau, C.; Loyer, M. Suicide and mental disorders: A case control study of young men. *Am. J. Psychiatry* **1994**, *151*, 1063–1068.
18. Hunt, I.M.; Kapur, N.; Robinson, J.; Shaw, J.; Flynn, S.; Bailey, H.; Meehan, J.; Bickley, H.; Burns, J.; Appleby, L.; et al. Suicide within 12 months of mental health service contact in different age and diagnostic groups: National clinical survey. *Br. J. Psychiatry* **2006**, *188*, 135–142. [CrossRef] [PubMed]
19. Tidemalm, D.; Elofsson, S.; Stefansson, C.-G.; Waern, M.; Runeson, B. Predictors of suicide in a community-based cohort of individuals with severe mental disorder. *Soc. Psychiatry Psychiatry Epidemiol.* **2005**, *40*, 595–600. [CrossRef] [PubMed]
20. Pompili, M.; Girardi, P.; Ruberto, A.; Tatarelli, R. Suicide in borderline personality disorder: A meta-analysis. *Nord. J. Psychiatry* **2005**, *59*, 319–324. [CrossRef] [PubMed]
21. McGirr, A.; Paris, J.; Lesage, A.; Renaud, J.; Turecki, G. Risk factors for suicide completion in borderline personality disorder: A case-control study of cluster B comorbidity and impulsive aggression. *J. Clin. Psychiatry* **2007**, *68*, 721–729. [CrossRef]
22. Zanarini, M.C.; Frankenburg, F.R.; Khera, G.S.; Bleichmar, J. Treatment histories of borderline inpatients. *Compr. Psychiatry* **2001**, *42*, 144–150. [CrossRef]
23. Goodman, M.; Roiff, T.; Oakes, A.H.; Paris, J. Suicidal risk and management in Borderline Personality Disorder. *Curr. Psychiatry Rep.* **2012**, *14*, 79–85. [CrossRef] [PubMed]
24. Turecki, G.; Brent, D. Suicide and suicidal behavior. *Lancet* **2016**, *387*, 19–25. [CrossRef]
25. Oldham, J.M.; Gabbard, G.O.; Goin, M.K.; Gunderson, J.; Soloff, P.; Spiegel, D.; Stone, M.; Phillips, K.A. Practice guideline for the treatment of Borderline Personality Disorder. *Am. J. Psychiatry* **2001**, *158*, 1–52.
26. Gunderson, J.G. *Borderline Personality Disorder: A Clinical Guide*, 2nd ed.; American Psychiatric Press: Washington, DC, USA, 2008.
27. Paris, J. *Half in Love with Death: The Meaning of Chronic Suicidality*; Laurence Erlbaum: Mahwah, NJ, USA, 2006.
28. Paris, J. *Stepped Care for Borderline Personality Disorder*; Academic Press: New York, NY, USA, 2017.
29. Linehan, M.M.; Armstrong, H.E.; Suarez, A.; Allmon, D.; Heard, H. Cognitive behavioral treatment of chronically parasuicidal borderline patients. *Arch. Gen. Psychiatry* **1991**, *48*, 1060–1064. [CrossRef] [PubMed]
30. Linehan, M.M.; Comtois, K.A.; Murray, A.M.; Brown, M.Z.; Gallop, R.J.; Heard, H.L.; Korslund, K.E.; Tutek, D.A.; Reyonolds, S.K.; Lindenboim, N. Two-year randomized controlled trial and follow-up of dialectical behavior therapy vs therapy by experts for suicidal behaviors and borderline personality disorder. *Arch. Gen. Psychiatry* **2006**, *63*, 757–766. [CrossRef] [PubMed]
31. Bateman, A.; Fonagy, P. Effectiveness of partial hospitalization in the treatment of borderline personality disorder: A randomized controlled trial. *Am. J. Psychiatry* **1999**, *156*, 1563–1569. [CrossRef] [PubMed]
32. Bateman, A.; Fonagy, P. Randomized controlled trial of out-patient mentalization-based treatment versus structured clinical management for borderline personality disorder. *Am. J. Psychiatry* **2009**, *166*, 1355–1364. [CrossRef] [PubMed]
33. Clarkin, J.F.; Levy, K.N.; Lenzenweger, M.F.; Kernberg, O.F. Evaluating three treatments for borderline personality disorder: A multiwave study. *Am. J. Psychiatry* **2007**, *164*, 1–8. [CrossRef]
34. Giesen-Bloo, J.; Van Dyck, R.; Spinhoven, P.; Van Tilburg, W.; Dirksen, C.; Van Asselt, T.; Kremers, I.; Nadort, M.; Arntz, A. Outpatient psychotherapy for borderline personality disorder: Randomized trial of schema-focused therapy vs. transference-focused psychotherapy. *Arch. Gen. Psychiatry* **2006**, *63*, 649–658. [CrossRef]

35. Davidson, K.; Norrie, J.; Tyrer, P.; Gumley, A.; Tata, P.; Murray, H. The effectiveness of cognitive behavior therapy for borderline personality disorder: Results from the borderline personality disorder study of cognitive therapy [BOSCOT] trial. *J. Personal. Disord.* **2006**, *20*, 450–465. [CrossRef]
36. Koenigsberg, H.W.; Harvey, P.D.; Mitropoulou, V.; Schmeidler, J.; New, A.S.; Goodman, M.; Silverman, J.M.; Serby, M.; Schopick, F.; Siever, L. Characterizing affective instability in borderline personality disorder. *Am. J. Psychiatry* **2002**, *159*, 784–788. [CrossRef]
37. Crowell, S.E.; Beauchaine, T.P.; Linehan, M.M. A biosocial developmental model of borderline personality: Elaborating and extending Linehan's theory. *Psychol. Bull.* **2009**, *135*, 495–510. [CrossRef]
38. Stoffers-Winterling, J.M.; Völlm, B.A.; Rücker, G.; Timmer, A.; Huband, N.; Lieb, K. Psychological interventions for borderline personality disorder. *Cochrane Library* **2012**. [CrossRef]
39. Cristea, I.A.; Gentilla, C.; Cotet, C.D.; Palomba, D.; Barbui, C.; Cuijpers, P. Efficacy of psychotherapies for Borderline Personality Disorder: A systematic review and meta-analysis. *JAMA Psychiatry* **2017**, *74*, 319–328. [CrossRef] [PubMed]
40. Zanarini, M.C. Psychotherapy of borderline personality disorder. *Acta Psychiatry Scand.* **2009**, *120*, 373–377. [CrossRef] [PubMed]
41. Binks, C.A.; Fenton, M.; McCarthy, L.; Lee, T.; Adams, C.E.; Duggan, C. Pharmacological interventions for people with borderline personality disorder. *Cochrane Database Syst. Rev.* **2012**, *1*, CD005653.
42. Crawford, M.; Sanatinia, R.; Barrett, B.M.; Cunningham, G. The clinical effectiveness and cost-effectiveness of lamotrigine in borderline personality disorder: A randomized placebo-controlled trial. *Am. J. Psychiatry* **2018**, *175*, 576–580. [CrossRef]
43. Black, D.W.; Zanarini, M.C.; Ronine, A.; Shaw, M.; Allen, J.; Schulz, S.C. Comparison of low and moderate dosages of extended-release quetiapine in Borderline Personality Disorder: A randomized, double-blind, placebo-controlled trial. *Am. J. Psychiatry* **2014**, *171*, 1174–1182. [CrossRef] [PubMed]
44. National Institutes of Clinical Excellence. Guidelines for the Treatment of Borderline Personality Disorder. 2009. Available online: http://www.nice.org.uk/guidance/index.jsp?action=byID&o=11651 (accessed on 10 May 2018).
45. Goldstein, R.B.; Black, D.W.; Nasrallah, A.; Winokur, G. The prediction of suicide. *Arch. Gen. Psychiatry* **1991**, *48*, 418–422. [CrossRef]
46. Pokorny, A.D. Prediction of suicide in psychiatric patients: Report of a prospective study. *Arch. Gen. Psychiatry* **1982**, *40*, 249–257. [CrossRef]
47. Schwartz, D.A.; Flinn, D.E.; Slawson, P.F. Treatment of the suicidal character. *Am. J. Psychiatry* **1974**, *28*, 194–207. [CrossRef]
48. Maltsberger, J.T. Calculated risk taking in the treatment of suicidal patients: Ethical and legal problems. *Death Stud.* **1994**, *18*, 439–452. [CrossRef]
49. Fowler, J.C.; Clapp, J.D.; Madan, A.; Allen, J.G.; Frueh, C.; Fonagy, P.; Oldham, J.M. A naturalistic longitudinal study of extended inpatient treatment for adults with borderline personality disorder: An examination of treatment response, remission and deterioration. *J. Affect. Disord.* **2018**, *235*, 323–331. [CrossRef] [PubMed]
50. Gutheil, T.G. Suicide and suit: Liability after self-destruction. In *Suicide and Clinical Practice*; Jacobs, D., Ed.; American Psychiatric Press: Washington, DC, USA, 1992; pp. 147–167.

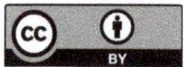

© 2019 by the author. Licensee MDPI, Basel, Switzerland. This article is an open access article distributed under the terms and conditions of the Creative Commons Attribution (CC BY) license (http://creativecommons.org/licenses/by/4.0/).

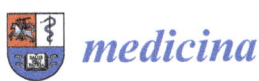

Review

The Role of Demoralization and Hopelessness in Suicide Risk in Schizophrenia: A Review of the Literature

Isabella Berardelli [1,*], Salvatore Sarubbi [2], Elena Rogante [2], Michael Hawkins [3], Gabriele Cocco [4], Denise Erbuto [1], David Lester [5] and Maurizio Pompili [1]

1. Department of Neurosciences, Mental Health and Sensory Organs, Suicide Prevention Center, Sant'Andrea Hospital, Sapienza University of Rome, 00185 Rome, Italy; denise.erbuto@uniroma1.it (D.E.); maurizio.pompili@uniroma1.it (M.P.)
2. Department of Psychology, Sapienza University of Rome, 00185 Rome, Italy; salvatore.sarubbi@uniroma1.it (S.S.); elena.rogante@gmail.com (E.R.)
3. Department of Psychiatry, University of Toronto, Toronto, ON M4B 1B4, Canada; michael.hawkins@mail.utoronto.ca
4. Faculty of Medicine and Psychology, Sapienza University of Rome, 00185 Rome, Italy; gabri.cocco84@hotmail.it
5. Psychology Program, Stockton University, Galloway, NJ 08205, USA; David.Lester@stockton.edu
* Correspondence: isabella.berardelli@uniroma1.it

Received: 26 March 2019; Accepted: 17 May 2019; Published: 23 May 2019

Abstract: *Background and Objectives:* Demoralization has been defined by hopelessness and helplessness attributable to a loss of purpose and meaning in life. Demoralization is a meaningful mental health concern, frequently associated with suicide risk in medical and psychiatric patients. The aim of this systematic review was to synthesize the recent empirical evidence on demoralization in patients with schizophrenia and to better understand the relationship between demoralization and suicide risk in patients with schizophrenia. *Methods:* A comprehensive literature search using key words and subject headings was performed following PRISMA guidelines with several bibliographic databases, resulting in the identification of 27 studies. *Results:* The findings suggested that demoralization is prevalent in patients with schizophrenia and supported the hypothesis that the association between depression and suicide is moderated by hopelessness. In clinical practice, it is important to recognize symptoms of demoralization using appropriate psychological tools to better understand the suffering of patients with schizophrenia and to implement suicide prevention programs.

Keywords: demoralization; schizophrenia; suicide risk

1. Introduction

Jerome Frank [1], more than forty years ago, defined demoralization as "a syndrome of existential distress occurring in patients with severe conditions that threaten life or integrity of being, such as physical illness or mental disorders." Demoralization is characterized by "feelings of impotence, isolation, and despair." Frank interpreted demoralization as an outcome caused by someone's failure to cope when faced with an event generally described as easy to manage [2]. In those who are demoralized, self-esteem suffers, and rejection is felt as a result of individuals believing they have failed to meet the expectations of others [1–3]. This highlights the salience that stressful events may have on the human psyche [4].

In more recent years, Irvin Yalom, an existential psychotherapist [5], noted how demoralization represents the outcome of a conflict between the individual and his personal existence. When a person is unable to face this conflict, demoralization can develop. Based on this, the definition of demoralization was subsequently enriched with new concepts [6], with the link between distress and subjective incompetence at the base of the construct of demoralization.

In the following years, several authors attempted to describe the demoralization syndrome. Fava et al. [7] used three diagnostic criteria for demoralization, including the failure of individuals to meet expectations set by themselves, those set by others, and their general inability to cope with demands. This results in feelings of helplessness, hopelessness, and a desire to give up. According to a psychosomatic perspective, demoralization is a predictor for the development of a medical illness [7].

A recent definition of demoralization was proposed by Kissane and Clarke [8,9] at the beginning of the 2000s. Demoralization was defined as a clinical entity characterized by symptoms such as existential distress, hopelessness, loss of meaning and purpose in life, a sense of being trapped, personal failure, and difficulty coping. Kissane focused on demoralization as a predictive variable for suicidal ideation in terminally ill patients [2]. Kissane described demoralization as an abnormal response characterized by two key aspects: loss of meaning in life and loss of hope. Considering that hopelessness is one of the most important predictors of suicide, patients with the demoralization syndrome may have a higher risk of suicide than patients without the demoralization syndrome [2].

The debate on demoralization as a syndrome is still controversial. The categorization of demoralization as an "abnormal response" has been criticized by different authors. Several authors emphasized that demoralization is a normal psychological response in patients affected by a medical illness [10] and compared demoralization to the Adjustment Disorders, described in DSM-5, or as a normal response to loss [11,12]. Furthermore, the main controversy centers on whether demoralization constitutes a syndrome of despair, distress, and hopelessness separate from depression. Kissane saw the concept of demoralization as a syndrome, contextualizing it on a spectrum where the end of this spectrum warrants a "psychiatric alert". Demoralization becomes clinically relevant when there is a significant loss of meaning and purpose in life, and suicidal thinking appears [13]. It has been argued that the critical feature distinguishing depression from demoralization is the presence or absence of anhedonia [14]. However, depression and anxiety are symptoms that are often present in the demoralization syndrome [8].

Although demoralization can occur in response to many distressing circumstances, much of the literature about demoralization focuses on people who have a terminal or severely disabling physical illness [15,16], but only a few studies have focused on psychiatric patients, such as patients with schizophrenia [17].

Patients with schizophrenia often die prematurely [18]. Though the lifetime risk for suicide for people with schizophrenia is estimated to be about 4.9% [19], up to 40% [20] of their premature mortality can be attributed to suicide and unnatural deaths. Several psychological features seem to contribute to suicide in this population, including hopelessness, recent loss or rejection, fear of further illness deterioration, awareness of their illness, loss of faith in treatment, post-psychotic depression, or failure in interpersonal relationships [21]. A number of clinical features have been associated with completed suicide in people with schizophrenia, including being young, male, Caucasian, and never married, and having good premorbid function and a history of substance abuse and suicide attempts [21,22]. Hopelessness, social isolation, and hospitalization are also important risk factors for completed suicide in individuals with schizophrenia. Among these features, hopelessness plays a large role in affecting the suicide risk of these patients. Higher hopelessness scores, regardless of the presence of only depressive symptoms, predicted a worse short-term outcome and worse global functioning, which are considered important risks factor for suicidal behavior [23]. Furthermore, a greater surveillance for suicide is required in the period after discharge from hospital and after periods of remission. Patients with schizophrenia usually experience hopelessness and demoralization after discharge from hospital which increases their suicide risk. During periods of remission, they can develop a painful awareness of their illness. At this point, their expectations contrast sharply with their declining functioning, leading to feelings of inadequacy, depression, and hopelessness. It has been suggested that hopelessness and greater insight are associated with current and lifetime risk of suicide [24].

Drake has described a demoralization syndrome in individuals with schizophrenia, in which repeated exacerbations of psychotic symptoms, functional deterioration, and a non-delusional awareness of the effects of the illness can lead to feelings of hopelessness, depression, and ultimately suicide [25].

In this view, premorbid adjustment and insight interact, resulting in demoralization and depression, potentially culminating in suicidal behavior. Interestingly, on the one hand, depression has been recognized as a major risk factor for suicide attempt among patients with schizophrenia [26]. On the other hand, depression is difficult to diagnose in patients with schizophrenia. In clinical practice, nonspecific sadness is more often observed than major depressive episodes. In the 1980s, Bartels and Drake [27] considered chronic demoralization to be a variable that predicted the risk of suicide in patients with schizophrenia. This hypothesis was then validated in several studies that have shown how the presence of depression, hopelessness, negative self-thoughts, anxiety, insomnia, self-devaluation, low self-esteem, and a feeling of guilt were strongly associated with a higher risk of suicide in patients with schizophrenia [21–28]. Research on this topic was then enriched with papers on patients with schizophrenia linking hopelessness with social and vocational dysfunction [29–31], suicide risk [25–32], avoidant coping [33,34], and stigma [35–37].

In line with the hypothesis that the demoralization syndrome and hopelessness are important risk factors for suicide in patients with schizophrenia, and on the basis that these two constructs are related to both patient insight and stigma, variables involved in suicide risk, we reviewed those studies investigating the presence of demoralization (and its constructs) and suicide, in patients with schizophrenia.

The principal aim of this review was to clarify the role of demoralization and hopelessness in affecting suicide risk in patients with schizophrenia. The second aim of this review paper was to better understand the complex relationship between demoralization and hopelessness, along with patient insight and stigma, and suicide risk in patients with schizophrenia.

2. Methods

We performed a systematic review of demoralization (according to a definition of demoralization that includes the inability to cope, helplessness, hopelessness, and low self-esteem) and suicidal risk in schizophrenia using MedLine, Excerpta Medica, PsycLit, PsycInfo, and Index Medicus search to identify all papers published between 1970 and 2018. The PRISMA statement for reporting systematic reviews was followed. Search terms used were: demoralization OR demoralization syndrome OR helplessness OR hopelessness AND suicide risk AND Schizophrenia, Psychosis. We first reviewed the titles and abstracts and applied the selection criteria outlined above with the exception of study design (Figure 1). Only articles published in English peer-reviewed journals were considered, and the articles were examined to for their relevance based on the inclusion criteria. Possible discrepancies between the reviewers with regard to inclusion criteria were resolved through consultation with the senior authors. In addition, reference lists were also examined. In the results section, we excluded case reports, meta-analyses, and systematic reviews, and studies that did not clearly report statistical analysis, diagnostic criteria, or the number of patients included. We found 27 articles on demoralization and schizophrenia that met these criteria and we discussed them in the two sections of the results (Clinical Studies included in qualitative synthesis). We have included three systematic reviews exclusively in the discussion section but not in the results section. The principal reviewer (IB) checked all items. Then, three reviewers independently inspected all citations of the studies identified by the search and grouped them according to topic.

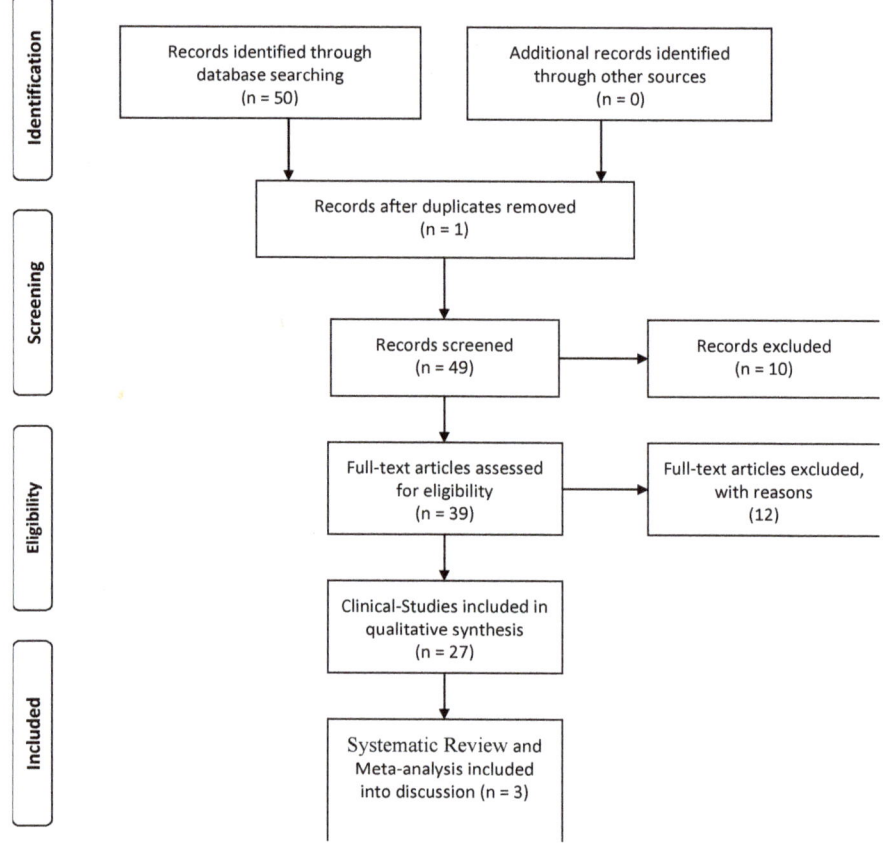

Figure 1. Flowchart of the search and selection process.

3. Results

3.1. Demoralization and Suicide Risk in Schizophrenia

Depressive features, including demoralization and hopelessness, are common in schizophrenia and are often intertwined with psychotic symptoms, becoming a significant mediator of disability and suicidality. Cotton et al. [38] interviewed 20 therapists who had clinically followed 20 patients with schizophrenia who completed suicide. These interviews indicated that the profile of the patients was of young men in their thirties with a chronic history of illness with exacerbations. From the interviews, it emerged that patients expressed hopelessness at the time of their suicide. The patients had a strong desire to escape through death, and most of them had a previous history of suicidal behavior. Cotton then showed how different clinical features resulted in guidelines for the treatment of these patients. For example, it is important to assess the patient's self-esteem, the protective function that psychosis may have in regard to suicide, and the importance of differentiating an inability to function from an unwillingness to function (i.e., unwillingness to share their thoughts of life and death or share the burden of despair resulting from their illness).

Drake et al. [39] examined risk factors for suicide in patients with schizophrenia, noting that the risk factors for suicide included demoralization and feelings of hopelessness and inadequacy. A few years later, the same authors investigated the clinical features of depression, hopelessness, and their relationship to major depressive episodes and suicides in 104 patients with schizophrenia, 15 of whom died by suicide [40]. Most patients (54%) endorsed "depressed mood", and 21% of these patients met DSM criteria for a depressive disorder. Although the presence of depressed mood increased their risk of suicide, the severity of depression did not increase the risk of suicide. In contrast, the development of hopelessness, in addition to depressed mood, significantly increased the probability of suicide. In absence of hopelessness, depressed patients with schizophrenia presented a similar risk for suicide to that of non-depressed patients with schizophrenia. Thus, these results suggest that hopelessness mediates the relationship between depression and suicide risk in patients with schizophrenia.

Data from a prospective community treatment study on suicide in patients with schizophrenia showed that the group of patients who died by suicide were younger, with an earlier onset of illness compared to patients who did not complete suicide, and suicide occurred very early in the course of illness [32]. Furthermore, hopelessness was a very discriminative feature between the two groups ($z = 3.27$, $p < 0.05$), and patients who completed suicide showed a significant increase in hopelessness and depression.

Fenton et al. [41] studied the relationship between positive and negative symptoms, illness subtype, and suicidal behavior in 187 patients with schizophrenia, 87 patients with schizoaffective disorder, 15 patients with schizophreniform disorder, and 33 patients with schizotypal personality disorder. The authors demonstrated that the progressive loss of social drive, the diminished capacity to experience affect, and an indifference toward the future may preclude the painful self-awareness associated with suicide.

Nordentoft et al. [42] investigated predictive factors for suicidal behavior in 321 patients with first-episode psychosis. Their results demonstrated that a suicide attempt was associated with younger age, depression, hopelessness, and hallucinations. Being female, reported hopelessness at baseline, the presence of hallucinations, and a suicide attempt reported at the initial interview were associated with a suicide attempt by the one-year follow up.

Kim et al. [43] enrolled 333 patients with schizophrenia to clarify the clinical role of hopelessness, insight, and cognitive dysfunction for suicide risk. They found that hopelessness was significantly higher in patients with lifetime suicidality and in those with current suicide risk compared to patients without history of suicidal behavior, thereby supporting the role of hopelessness as a predictor of the lifetime risk of suicide.

Montross et al. [44] examined the prevalence of suicidal behavior in 132 patients with schizophrenia. Depression and hopelessness were significantly higher in the group with suicidal ideation. Predictive features for current suicidal ideation included depression, hopelessness, gender, general psychopathology, and the presence of a past suicide attempt. They also found that hopelessness and a past history of suicide attempts were the only variables associated with current suicidal ideation.

Restifo et al. [45] tested the demoralization hypothesis as an independent risk factor for suicidal behaviors in 164 patients, 115 of whom had a diagnosis of schizophrenia and 49 a diagnosis of schizoaffective disorder. The sample was divided in two groups: patients with a history of a previous suicide attempt ($N = 59$) and patients without a history of previous suicide attempts ($N = 105$). The authors observed that premorbid functioning and insight were associated with more depressive symptoms. Furthermore, cognitive symptoms of depression (poor concentration, indecisiveness, forgetfulness) and subclinical symptoms of depression were linked with past suicide attempts, while hopelessness predicted current and lifetime risk of suicide among these patients with schizophrenia. In support of these results, a case-control study [46] confirmed that a history of suicide attempts, hopelessness, and self-devaluation were the three variables that had the strongest association with completed suicide in patients with schizophrenia.

More recently Klonsky, et al. [47], in a 10-year longitudinal study of 414 patients with first-admission psychosis, clarified the relationship between hopelessness and suicide attempt. Both hopelessness and recent suicide attempts were assessed at multiple time-points. The results demonstrated that hopelessness at baseline predicted a suicide attempt during the subsequent 10 years independent of the presence of depression.

A few studies have investigated the association between self-esteem and suicide risk in patients with schizophrenia [48] (Table 1). Tarrier et al. [49] examined 59 patients with recent onset schizophrenia, reporting that greater hopelessness (odds ratio (OR) 1.22) and a longer duration of illness (OR 1.13) increased the risk of suicide in these patients. Hopelessness was associated with higher negative self-evaluation and social isolation, while negative self-evaluation was associated with self-criticism and negative symptoms. Acosta et al. [50], in a study of 60 patients with schizophrenia showed that negative cognitions about the psychiatric diagnosis were associated with depressive symptoms and hopelessness. Interestingly, negative cognition did not differ in patients with and without a history of previous suicide attempts. Yoo et al. [51] studied 87 patients with schizophrenia, of whom 20 (23.0%) had a history of suicide attempts. Their results revealed that patients with a history of suicide attempts had significantly higher scores on the Beck Depression Inventory ($p = 0.036$) and on the Korean version of the Internalized Stigma of Mental Illness scale ($p = 0.009$), and significantly lower scores on the Rosenberg Self-Esteem Scale ($p = 0.001$), demonstrating that low self-esteem represents a psychological feature of those who attempt suicide, thereby increasing their risk of suicide.

Table 1. Demoralization and Suicide Risk in Schizophrenia.

Authors	Purpose	Measures	Results/Discussion
Drake et al. (1984)	Risk factors for suicide in patients with schizophrenia N = 104 (15 clinical vs. 89 controls; all met DSM-III diagnostic criteria for Schizophrenia)	3d edition of the Diagnostic and Statistical Manual of Mental Disorders from the American Psychiatric Association (DSM-III)	Depressed mental status is more frequently observed in suicide group vs. non-suicide group (80% vs. 48%; $p < 0.01$).
Cotton et al. (1985)	Psychotherapy of suicidal schizophrenic patients. N = 20 (schizophrenia)	Semi-structured interviews	Patients with schizophrenia reported hopelessness and a strong desire to escape through death at the time of suicide. It is important to assess self-esteem, the presence of psychosis, and distinguish inability to function from unwillingness to function
Drake & Cotton (1986)	DSM-III depressive symptoms vs. hopelessness in schizophrenic suicides and non-suicides patients N = 104 (15 = s; 89 = n-s)	3d edition of the Diagnostic and Statistical Manual of Mental Disorders from the American Psychiatric Association (DSM-III); Beck Hopelessness Scale (BHS)	Suicide ideas, depressive mood, and hopelessness rather than depression increases risk of suicide (respectively 87%, 80%, and 67% vs. 33% of depression in suicide sample); $p < 0.01$
Cohen et al. (1990)	Suicide in long-term treatment schizophrenia. N = 122 (67.2% male) with Schizophrenia, schizoaffective disorder (research diagnostic criteria), or schizotypal personality disorder (DSM-III)	Symptom Checklist 90-R (SCL-90-R); Brief Psychiatric Rating Scale (BPRS); Self-report measure of satisfaction	Baseline SCL-90-R scores for: hopelessness (6.30 vs. 2.96), hostility (3.53 vs. 1.63), depression (5.89 vs. 3.52), paranoid ideation (4.51 vs. 2.71), and obsessive-compulsive (3.73 vs. 2.23) were very discriminative between suicides (N = 8) and non-suicides (N = 74)

Table 1. Cont.

Authors	Purpose	Measures	Results/Discussion
Fenton et al. (1997)	Suicidality in schizophrenia and its relationship with subtypes N = 322 (schizophrenia n = 187; schizoaffective disorder n = 87; schizophreniform disorder N = 15; schizotypal personality disorder n = 33)	3d edition of the Diagnostic and Statistical Manual of Mental Disorders from the American Psychiatric Association (DSM-III); Positive and Negative Symptoms Scale (PANSS); self-report interviews	Negative symptoms: blunted affect ($p = 0.03$), poverty of speech ($p = 0.02$), stereotyped thinking ($p = 0.005$), and only one of positive symptoms (grandiosity ($p < 0.05$)) were correlated with suicide behavior.
Nordentoft et al. (2002)	Suicidal behavior and treatment in first-episode schizophrenia (FEP) N = 341 (FEP disorder); attempts reported at baseline (N = 321); attempts during first year of treatment (N = 275) Diagnosis: schizophrenia, schizotypal disorder, delusional disorder, acute or transient psychosis, schizoaffective psychosis, induced psychosis, or unspecific non-organic psychosis according to ICD–10	Schedules for Clinical Assessment in Neuropsychiatry (SCAN 2.0), Scale for the Assessment of Negative Symptoms (SANS), Scale for the Assessment of Positive Symptoms (SAPS)	Baseline period: being male ($p = 0.001$) and suicidal plans the week prior ($p = 0.001$) were significant predictors of suicide; Follow up period: being male ($p = 0.002$), suicidal plans the week prior ($p < 0.001$), and previous suicide attempts ($p = 0.001$) were significantly associated with suicide. There was a weak association between hopelessness and suicide in the integrated treatment's group one year after treatment compared to the standard treatment's group ($p < 0.01$)
Kim et al. (2002)	Hopelessness, insight, cognitive dysfunction, and suicidality in schizophrenia N = 333 (schizophrenia)	Schedule for Affective Disorders and Schizophrenia (SADS), Hamilton Depression Rating Scale (HDRS), Brief Psychiatric Rating Scale (BPRS)	Regression analysis predicted Hopelessness as the most important predictor of current and lifetime suicidality ($\beta = 0.41$, $p = 0.0001$; $\beta = 0.35$, $p = 0.01$, respectively). Further, insight and substance abuse were predictors for lifetime and current suicidality ($p = 0.001$ and $p = 0.004$; $p = 0.001$ and $p = 0.033$, respectively).
Tarrier et al. (2004)	Factors (self-esteem, relatives' expressed emotions, demographic, social, clinical) associated with suicidal ideation and/or previous suicide attempts as proxy measures of suicide risk N = 59 (DSM-IV diagnosis of recent onset schizophrenia)	4d edition of the Diagnostic and Statistical Manual of Mental Disorders from the American Psychiatric Association (DSM-IV); Modified Self-Evaluation and Social Support for Schizophrenia (SESS-sv); Positive and Negative Symptoms Scale (PANSS); Beck Depression Inventory (BDI); Beck Hopelessness Scale (BHS); Insight Scale (IS)	Greater hopelessness (OR 1.22) and longer duration of illness (OR 1.13) increase suicide risk. Hopelessness was also associated with higher negative self-evaluation and social isolation.

Table 1. Cont.

Authors	Purpose	Measures	Results/Discussion
Ran et al. (2005)	Suicide attempters' (N = 38) vs. non-attempters' (N = 472) clinical features. N = 510 (schizophrenia)	Screening schedule for Psychosis, Present State Examination, Chinese version (PSE-9), Social Disability Screening Schedule (SDSS), General Psychiatric Interview Schedule and Summary Form	Hopelessness and depressed mood were present in 60.5% of the patients with a history of lifetime suicide attempt ($p < 0.001$).
Montross et al. (2008)	Prevalence and correlates of suicide in 40-year-old and older schizophrenic patients N = 132 (schizophrenia spectrum disorder and concurrent depressive symptoms)	SCID, Beck Scale for Suicidal Ideation (BSSI), Hamilton Depression Rating Scale (HAM-D), Calgary Depression Rating Scale (CDRS), Positive and Negative Symptoms Scale (PANSS), Clinical Global Impression Scale (CGI), Cumulative Illness Rating Scale-Geriatrics version C(IRS-G), Beck Hopelessness Scale (BHS)	Hopelessness rated by BHS (5.8; $p = 0.001$), and level of depression rated by HAM-D (13; $p = 0.000$) and CDR (6.4; $p = 0.001$) significantly differentiated the suicidal ideation and non-suicidal ideation groups.
Restifo et al. (2009)	Demoralization model (premorbid adjustment x insight) N = 164 (schizophrenia, N = 115; schizoaffective, N = 49)	Diagnostic Interview of Genetic Studies (DIGS), Premorbid Adjustment Scale (PAS)	Interaction between premorbid adjustment and insight did not significantly predict suicide attempt ($p = 0.88, p = 0.91$)
Pompili et al. (2009)	Understanding suicide risk in 20 patients with schizophrenia who died by suicide vs. C 20 controls	Beck Hopelessness Scale (BHS)	Hopelessness (OR = 51.00; 95%CI = 7.56–343.72) was a risk factor for suicide
Klonsky et al. (2012)	Longitudinal relationship of hopelessness and attempted suicide in DSM-III-R psychotic disorders N = 414	3d edition of the Diagnostic and Statistical Manual of Mental Disorders from the American Psychiatric Association DSM-III-R; Beck Hopelessness Scale (BHS); Hamilton Depression Rating Scale (HAM-D)	Hopelessness in psychotic disorders provides information about suicide risk. In comparison to non-psychotic population, even relatively modest levels of hopelessness increase risk for suicide in psychotic patients.
Acosta et al. (2012)	Relationship between schizophrenic patients' cognitions about their illness and past suicidal behaviors Relationship between patients' beliefs about the illness with potential mediators of suicidal behaviors such as depressive symptoms, hopelessness, and insight N = 60 (ICD-10 diagnosis of schizophrenia)	International Classification of Diseases 10th Revision); (ICD-10); Calgary Depression Scale (CDS); Beck Hopelessness Scale (BHS);	Negative appraisals were associated with hopelessness and depressive symptoms (negative expectations and stigma showed the strongest associations). No differences between patients with and without past suicidal behaviors

Table 1. Cont.

Authors	Purpose	Measures	Results/Discussion
Fulginiti & Brekke (2015)	Association between discrepancy factors (self-esteem and quality of life) and suicidal ideation in DSM-IV schizophrenia spectrum disorders N = 162	4d edition of the Diagnostic and Statistical Manual of Mental Disorders (DSM-IV); Extended Version of the Brief Psychiatric Rating Scale (BPRS-E); Subjective Well-being under Neuroleptic Treatment scale (SWL); Index for Self-Esteem (ISE); Medical Outcomes Study Social Support Survey (MOS-SSS); Survey); RFS (Role Functioning Scale)	QoL and self-esteem added value to predicting suicidal ideation beyond clinical and demographic factors. Self-esteem mediates the relationship between QoL and suicidal ideation.
Yoo et al. (2015)	Associations between suicidality and self-esteem in patients with schizophrenia according to DSM-IV N = 87 (20 attempted suicide)	4d edition of the Diagnostic and Statistical Manual of Mental Disorders (DSM-IV); Positive and Negative Symptoms Scale (PANSS); Beck Depression Inventory (BDI); Beck Hopelessness Scale (BHS); Rosenberg Self-Esteem Scale (SES); Korean version of the Internalized Stigma of Mental Illness Scale (K-ISMI)	Patients with a history of suicide attempt had significantly higher scores on BDI ($p = 0.036$) and K-ISMI ($p = 0.009$) and significantly lower scores on SES ($p = 0.001$).

Five hundred and ten individuals with schizophrenia were studied by Ran et al. [52] with the aim of identifying clinical variables that could discern between patients with a history of suicide attempts and those without a history of suicide attempts. Of the 510 patients, 60.5% of patients that attempted suicide endorsed depressive symptoms and hopelessness. The suicide attempters also had more auditory hallucinations, delusions, and positive symptoms and presence of lifetime hopelessness.

3.2. Demoralization, Insight, and Stigma in Schizophrenia

How depression, demoralization, hopelessness, positive and negative symptoms, illness subtype, and suicidal tendency relate to one another in patients with schizophrenia is poorly understood but of great clinical relevance. Several studies have highlighted the link between high levels of insight, low self-esteem, and the quality of life [53,54] (Table 2). Patients with psychiatric illnesses experience discrimination, less life satisfaction, stigma, and feel demoralized and rejected by others [55]. Recent research has suggested that self-stigma results in reduced self-esteem, depression, and anxiety and hinders recovery [56,57]. In a cross-sectional study on 85 patients with schizophrenia receiving maintenance therapy, Birchwood et al. [58] investigated the relationship between depression, the acceptance or rejection of mental illness, the perceived controllability of illness and the acceptance of cultural stereotypes. Twenty-nine per cent of the patients with schizophrenia were considered 'depressed' using the cut-off point of 15 on the Beck Depression Inventory (BDI).

Table 2. Demoralization, insight, and stigma in schizophrenia.

Authors	Purpose	Measures	Results/Discussion
Birchwood et al. (1993)	Relationship between depression and acceptance or rejection of mental illness and perceived controllability of illness in chronic psychosis N = 84 (49 schizophrenia, 35 manic-depressive disorder)	Beck Depression Inventory (BDI); Personal Beliefs about Illness Questionnaire (PBIQ); Crown Self-Esteem Scale; degree of acceptance of two statements regarding acceptance or rejection of mental illness label	Patients' perception of controllability of their illness powerfully discriminated depressed from non-depressed psychotic patients. Label acceptance was not associated with depression, low self-esteem, or unemployment.
Aguilar et al. (1997)	Hopelessness in first-episode psychotic patients in 96 neuroleptic-naive psychotic patients (49 schizophrenic patients and 47 other non-affective psychotic patients)	Hopelessness Scale (HS)	High HS scores at baseline predicted poor short-term outcome in patients with schizophrenia, as evidenced by worse global functioning at the 12-month follow-up.
Carrol et al. (2004)	Explores the level of insight in patients with schizophrenia and its relationship to symptoms and history of violence. Relationship between the insight's dimensions of "compliance" and "awareness of illness" and hopelessness N = 28 (DSM-IV diagnosis of schizophrenia)	4d edition of the Diagnostic and Statistical Manual of Mental Disorders (DSM-IV); Beck Hopelessness Scale (BHS); Positive and Negative Symptoms Scale (PANSS);	Awareness of illness ($p = 0.028$), but not compliance with treatment, was positively correlated with level of hopelessness.
Lysaker et al. (2004)	Explores two aspects of hope (expectations of the future and motivation to persist), neurocognition, personality, symptoms, and social functioning in post-acute phase of schizophrenia N = 52 (39 DSM-IV diagnosis of schizophrenia; 13 DSM-IV diagnosis of schizoaffective disorder)	4d edition of the Diagnostic and Statistical Manual of Mental Disorders (DSM-IV); Positive and Negative Symptoms Scale (PANSS); Hopkins Verbal Learning Test (HVLT); Wisconsin Card Sorting Test (WCST); (NEO Five-Factor Inventory (NEO); Vocabulary; Beck Hopelessness Scale (BHS); Quality of Life Scale (QOL)	Neuroticism, verbal memory, and income were each related to expectations of the future. Neuroticism and social isolation were related to motivational hope. Positive and negative symptoms were unrelated to either form of hopelessness.

Table 2. *Cont.*

Authors	Purpose	Measures	Results/Discussion
White et al. (2007)	Relationship between psychiatric symptoms levels, beliefs about illness and hopelessness N = 100 (DSM-IV diagnosis of schizophrenia)	4d edition of the Diagnostic and Statistical Manual of Mental Disorders (DSM-IV); Personal Beliefs about Illness Questionnaire (PBIQ); Extended Version of the Brief Psychiatric Rating Scale (BPRS); Scale for the Assessment of Negative Symptoms (SANS); Beck Hopelessness Scale (BHS);	There were significant differences between the hopeless and non-hopeless participants on PBIQ, SANS, and BPRS. CDSS score, "humiliating need to be marginalized" PBIQ subscale and BPRS score contributed significantly (60% of the variance) to hopelessness scores.
Cavelti et al. (2012)	Mechanisms underlying the association of insight, depressive symptoms, and protective factors in patients with DSM-IV diagnosis of schizophrenic spectrum disorders N = 142	4d edition of the Diagnostic and Statistical Manual of Mental Disorders (DSM-IV); Scale to Assess Unawareness of Mental Disorder (SUMD); Beck Depression Inventory (BDI-II); Subjective Well-being under Neuroleptic Treatment scale (SWN); Illness Perception Questionnaire for Schizophrenia (IPQS);	Higher levels of insight and psychotic symptoms were associated with more depressive symptoms. Participants' perception of their illness as chronic and disabling mediates the relationship between insight and depressive symptoms. The association of insight and depressive symptoms was less pronounced in patients with positive recovery attitude
Cavelti et al. (2012)	Investigates self-stigma both as a moderator and as a mediator variable in the relationship between insight and demoralization in patients with DSM-IV diagnosis of schizophrenic spectrum disorder N = 145	4d edition of the Diagnostic and Statistical Manual of Mental Disorders (DSM-IV); Scale to Assess Unawareness of Mental Disorder (SUMD); Beck Depression Inventory (BDI); Subjective Well-being under Neuroleptic Treatment scale (SWN); Self-Stigma of Mental Illness Scale (SSMIS);	The association of insight and demoralization was stronger as self-stigma increased, confirming self-stigma as a moderator. Self-stigma also partially mediates the positive relationship between insight and demoralization. Demoralization fully mediates the adverse associations of self-stigma with psychotic symptoms and global functioning
Boursier et al. (2013)	Demoralization in psychotic patients N = 55 (schizophrenic disorder)	Positive and Negative Symptoms Scale (PANSS), Beck Hopelessness Scale (BHS), Poor quality of life (SqOL)	94% of the sample was found to be demoralized. Demoralization correlates with positive symptoms ($p = 0.016$), depression ($p < 0.001$), despair ($p = 0.015$), suicidality ($p < 0.01$), and poor quality of life ($p = 0.007$).

Table 2. *Cont.*

Authors	Purpose	Measures	Results/Discussion
Vass et al. (2015)	Impact of stigma on symptomatic and subjective recovery from psychosis (currently and longitudinally). Investigates whether self-esteem and hopelessness mediate the association between stigma and outcomes N = 80	International Classification of Diseases 10th Revision (ICD-10); Beck Hopelessness Scale (BHS); Questionnaire about the Process of Recovery (QPR); Positive and Negative Symptoms Scale (PANSS)	Stigma predicted both symptomatic and subjective recovery. Hopelessness and self-esteem mediated the effect of stigma on symptomatic and subjective recovery. At the follow-up, stigma predicted recovery and symptoms.
Wartelsteiner et al. (2016)	Examines the correlation of resilience, self-esteem, hopelessness, and psychopathology with quality of life N = 129 (52 DSM-IV diagnosis of schizophrenia; 77 healthy controls)	4d edition of the Diagnostic and Statistical Manual of Mental Disorders	Patients with schizophrenia had lower levels of QoL, resilience, self-esteem, and hope than healthy control subjects. In these patients, QoL correlated moderately with resilience, self-esteem, and hopelessness and weakly with symptoms (negative correlation with depression and positive symptoms)
Touriño et al. (2018)	Assesses prevalence of internalized stigma in patients with ICD-10 diagnosis of schizophrenia who attend psychosocial rehabilitation programs. Investigate the relationship between internalized stigma and sociodemographic, general clinical, psychopathologic, psychological, and suicidal behaviour variables in schizophrenic patients N = 71	ICD-10; ISMI; RSES; SUMD; BHS; CGI-SCH; CDS; SCS	Stigma was associated with higher prevalence of suicidal ideation, a higher number of suicide attempts, higher current suicidal risk, worse self-compassion, higher self-esteem, higher scores on depression, higher prevalence of depression, and higher hopelessness. Hopelessness and the existence of depression were independently associated with internalized stigma

The relationship between hopelessness and global functioning was investigated by Aguilar et al. [59] in first-episode psychosis patients. They found that patients with first-episode schizophrenia had higher levels of hopelessness than non-schizophrenia patients, and that higher hopelessness scores predicted worse global functioning at a one-year follow-up in patients with psychosis. In a cross-sectional study, Carroll et al. [60] explored the relationship between hopelessness and level of insight in 28 forensic patients with schizophrenia, testing the hypothesis that insight domains of 'compliance with treatment' and 'awareness of illness', as evaluated by the Schedule for Assessment of Insight (SAI), would be positively correlated with hopelessness. They showed that awareness of illness, but not compliance with the treatment, was positively correlated with level of hopelessness (i.e., patients who had a poor awareness of their illness generally had more hope for their future).

Lysaker et al. [61] investigated whether expectations about the future and motivation to persist (two aspects of hope) were correlated with neurocognitive patterns, personality, symptoms, and social functioning among 52 patients in a post-acute phase of schizophrenia. The authors suggested that both these aspects of hope were linked to lesser levels of stigma, fewer symptoms of schizophrenia, lesser anxiety, and lesser preference for avoidant forms of coping, emphasizing how different aspects of stigma are possibly linked to different domains of hope.

White et al. [62], in a study on 100 patients with schizophrenia, investigated the psychological features of non-hopeless patients (including personal beliefs about illness) and versus hopeless patients. Of the total sample, 25% of patients reported severe hopelessness, and hopelessness correlated significantly with "entrapment", "loss of autonomy", and "attribution: of self vs. illness" (the extent to which the individual believes that the origins of the illness lie in their personal psyche), using subscales of the Personal Beliefs about Illness Questionnaire (PBIQ). White et al. concluded that, although depression and hopelessness scores are highly correlated, the abovementioned aspects of a patient's personal belief about their illness were all independently associated with hopelessness after controlling for depression.

Cavelti et al. [63] demonstrated that the association between insight and demoralization is mediated by the participants' perception of their mental illness as being chronic, disabling, and out of control. The same authors [64] confirmed, in a study of 145 outpatients with schizophrenia, that the relationship between insight and demoralization was stronger as self-stigma increased, that is, patients with high insight tended to be more demoralized as a result, in part, of their increased likelihood of experiencing self-stigma in relation to their mental illness. In the same study, self-stigma also partially mediated the positive relationship between insight and demoralization, that is, the impact of insight on demoralization diminished after self-stigma was included in the regression equation. Moreover, demoralization fully mediated the adverse associations of self-stigma with psychotic symptoms and global functioning (i.e., higher levels of psychotic symptoms and lower levels of functioning were correlated with higher levels of demoralization).

Boursier et al. [65] investigated the presence of demoralization in 55 patients with schizophrenia, demonstrating that more than 94% of these patients experienced demoralization. The degree of demoralization was correlated with the intensity of positive symptoms, depression, despair, suicidality, poor quality of life, and low self-esteem.

A recent study by Wartelsteiner et al. [66] found that schizophrenia patients had significantly lower quality of life (QoL), resilience, self-esteem, and hope compared to healthy control subjects, highlighting the complex nature of QoL in patients suffering from schizophrenia and the importance of enhancing resilience and self-esteem and diminishing hopelessness and psychopathological features in patients with schizophrenia.

Recently Tourino et al. [67], in a sample of 71 outpatients with a diagnosis of schizophrenia, found that, in 21.1% of these patients, stigma was associated with suicidal ideation, a higher number of suicide attempts, higher current suicidal risk, worse self-compassion, higher scores for depression, a higher prevalence of depression, and higher levels of hopelessness.

4. Discussion

In this review, we have shown a clinical overlap between symptoms of demoralization and schizophrenia. Currently, it is estimated that the prevalence of depressive disorders in schizophrenia is around 40% [68,69] and the presence of depression is correlated with poorer outcomes in schizophrenia [70,71]. Bartels and Drake [27] suggested that depressive symptoms in schizophrenia included depressive symptoms secondary to organic factors, "nonorganic" depression intrinsic to the acute psychotic episode, and depressive symptoms that are not associated with the acute psychotic episode, such as symptoms associated with the prodromal, post-psychotic interval, as well as those symptoms that resemble depression that may represent negative symptoms of schizophrenia. Based on the results of this review, we suggest including the *Demoralization Syndrome* among the depressive syndromes in schizophrenia.

The demoralization syndrome can be differentiated from depression. In patients with chronic medical illness and in patients with psychiatric disorders, disability, bodily disfigurement, fear of loss of dignity, social isolation, feelings of greater dependency on others, and the perception of being a burden may predispose patients to develop symptoms of demoralization. Furthermore, patients with the demoralization syndrome, composed of the sense of impotence and helplessness, could progress to a desire to die by suicide. The research reviewed demonstrated clearly that suicide risk is associated with hopelessness and depression [21], and that suicidal intent in psychiatric inpatients correlates more strongly with hopelessness than with depression [72]. The results of this paper further support the argument for distinguishing demoralization syndrome and its constructs from clinical depression in patients affected by schizophrenia [9].

Previous research has shown that the patients with schizophrenia who are at a higher risk to die by suicide are those who are young, male, Caucasian, never married, with good premorbid function, post-psychotic depression, and with a history of substance abuse and suicide attempts. Furthermore, hopelessness, social isolation, hospitalization, deteriorating health with a high level of premorbid functioning, recent loss or rejection, limited external support, and family stress are considered important risk factors in patients with schizophrenia who die by suicide. How depression, demoralization, hopelessness, positive and negative symptoms, illness subtype, and suicidal tendency evolved in relation to each other in patients with schizophrenia is poorly understood but of clinical relevance. As shown above, several studies have highlighted the link between high levels of insight and low self-esteem and quality of life [52,53]. Patients with psychiatric illnesses experience discrimination, less life satisfaction, stigma, and feel demoralized and rejected by others [54].

The research review above shows how demoralization is frequently present in patients with schizophrenia and its significant association with suicide risk. Furthermore, hopelessness has been found to predict current and lifetime suicidality among patients with schizophrenia, independently of a diagnosis of major depression [43–71], emphasizing the importance of assessing demoralization symptoms in psychiatric patients to better evaluate suicide risk in clinical settings.

This review supports the hypothesis that the association between depression and suicide is moderated by hopelessness. Hopelessness may operate as a powerful potentiating variable, as demonstrated by the evidence showing that depression becomes a predictor of suicide only in the presence of hopelessness. Furthermore, the results of our review, which demonstrated the relationship between demoralization, insight, and stigma in patients affected by schizophrenia, suggest that demoralization may add valuable information about clinically relevant psychological distress in the context of psychiatric diseases. Self-insight may exert its effect on suicide risk through increasing demoralization, rather than through a direct impact on suicidal behavior. Studies in this field suggested that insight may represent a risk factor for suicide in patients with schizophrenia and this association appears to be mediated by other variables, such as depression and, above all, hopelessness. Further studies are required to analyze this issue in depth, given the crucial implications that it may have on the development of a model for suicide prevention in schizophrenia.

Limitations

When interpreting the results of this review, several limitations should be considered. First, all reviews of research are retrospective and, therefore, are subject to bias. Second, we selected only articles in English, omitting relevant articles in other languages from our review. Third, we did not examine the role of gender on suicide risk. Fourth, it was not always simple to apply the concept of "demoralization" retroactively to studies that did not specifically set out to study it, for example ones that look at "hopelessness" or "helplessness". Moreover, given this difficulty, the division of the two sub-chapters of the result section can sometimes seem confusing. Specifically, we included in the first section the studies that presented the main focus on suicidal risk and in the second chapter the studies that mainly considered demoralization, insight, stigma, and quality of life in patients affected by schizophrenia.

Finally, not all the studies reviewed in this paper distinguished completed suicide from attempted suicide. Suicide attempters and completers with schizophrenia appear to represent two overlapping but distinct groups, with different clinical and demographic profiles.

5. Conclusions

Despite increased screening for depression in clinical settings, demoralization symptoms in patients with schizophrenia are often either missed or dismissed by clinicians. This is at least in part because of the difficulty of distinguishing between symptoms of a concurrent mood disorder and those of the schizophrenia syndrome itself, in which disturbed affect and difficulty expressing emotions are central negative symptoms. Our results suggest that, in clinical practice, it is important to recognize the symptoms of demoralization, in particular hopelessness, using appropriate psychological tools in order to better approach the suffering of our patients and implement suicide prevention programs in patients with schizophrenia. Identifying specific subgroups of patients with schizophrenia with different suicide risk profiles, including the presence of demoralization symptoms, is an important goal for future research. Furthermore, in clinical practice, clinicians should definitely focus on the degree of insight in their clients in order to evaluate the suicidal risk, through a careful clinical evaluation and through the use of appropriate tools that evaluate and prevent suicidal risk.

Author Contributions: I.B. wrote the manuscript, S.S., E.R., M.H., G.C. and D.E. contributed to the collection of articles, D.L. corrected and reviewed the article. M.P. provided the original idea and the intellectual impetus.

Funding: This research received no external funding.

Acknowledgments: No Acknowledgments.

Conflicts of Interest: The authors declare no conflict of interest.

References

1. Frank, J.D. Psychotherapy: The restoration of morale. *Am. J. Psychiatry* **1974**, *131*, 271–274. [CrossRef]
2. Robinson, S.; Kissane, D.W.; Brooker, J.; Burney, S. A Review of the construct of demoralization: History, definitions, and future direction for palliative care. *Am. J. Hos. Pall. Med.* **2014**, *33*, 93–101. [CrossRef]
3. Frank, J.D. *Persuasion and Healing: A Comparative Study of Psychotherapy*, 2nd ed.; JHU Press: Baltimore, MD, USA, 1993.
4. Frank, J.D. The role of hope in psychotherapy. *Int. J. Psychiatry* **1968**, *5*, 383–395. [PubMed]
5. Yalom, I.D. *The Yalom Reader: Selections from the Work of a Master Therapist and Storyteller*; Basic Books: New York, NY, USA, 1996.
6. De Figueiredo, J.M.; Frank, J.D. Subjective incompetence, the clinical hallmark of demoralization. *Compr. Psychiatry* **1982**, *23*, 353–363. [CrossRef]
7. Fava, G.A.; Freyberger, H.J.; Bech, P.; Christodoulou, G.; Sensky, T.; Theorell, T.; Wise, T.N. Diagnostic criteria for use in psychosomatic research. *Psychother. Psychosom.* **1995**, *63*, 1–8. [CrossRef]
8. Kissane, D.W.; Clarke, D.M.; Street, A.F. Demoralization syndrome: A relevant psychiatric diagnosis for palliative care. *J. Palliat. Care* **2001**, *17*, 12–21. [CrossRef]
9. Clarke, D.M.; Kissane, D.W. Demoralization: Its phenomenology and importance. *Aust. N. Z. J. Psychiatry* **2002**, *36*, 733–742. [CrossRef]
10. Sansone, R.A.; Sansone, L.A. Demoralization in patients with medical illness. *Psychiatry* **2010**, *7*, 42. [PubMed]
11. Slavney, P.R. Diagnosing demoralization in consultation psychiatry. *Psychosomatics* **1999**, *40*, 325–329. [CrossRef]
12. Angelino, A.F.; Treisman, G.J. Major depression and demoralization in cancer patients: Diagnostic and treatment considerations. *Support Care Cancer* **2001**, *9*, 344. [CrossRef] [PubMed]
13. Kissane, D.W. Distress, demoralization and depression in palliative care. *Curr Ther.* **2000**, *41*, 14–19.
14. Pasquini, M.; Berardelli, I.; Biondi, M. Ethiopathogenesis of depressive disorders. Clinical practice and epidemiology in mental health. *Clin. Pract. Epidemiol. Ment. Health* **2014**, *10*, 166–171. [CrossRef] [PubMed]

15. Tecuta, L.; Tomba, E.; Grandi, S.; Fava, G.A. Demoralization: A systematic review on its clinical characterization. *Psychol. Med.* **2015**, *45*, 673–691. [CrossRef] [PubMed]
16. Fava, G.A.; Cosci, F.; Sonino, N. Current psychosomatic practice. *Psychother. Psychosom.* **2017**, *86*, 13–30. [CrossRef]
17. Grassi, L.; Mangelli, L.; Fava, G.A.; Grandi, S.; Ottolini, F.; Porcelli, P.; Rafanelli, C.; Rigatelli, M.; Sonino, N. Psychosomatic characterization of adjustment disorders in the medical setting: Some suggestions for DSM-V. *J. Affect. Disord.* **2007**, *101*, 251–254. [CrossRef]
18. Nordentoft, M.; Wahlbeck, K.; Hallgren, J.; Westman, J.; Osby, U.; Alinaghizadeh, H.; Gissler, M.; Laursen, T.M. Excess mortality, causes of death and life expectancy in 270,770 patients with recent onset of mental disorders in Denmark, Finland and Sweden. *PLoS ONE* **2013**, *8*, e55176. [CrossRef]
19. Palmer, B.A.; Pankratz, V.S.; Bostwick, J.M. The lifetime risk of suicide in Schizophrenia: A reexamination. *Arch. Gen. Psychiatry* **2005**, *62*, 247–253. [CrossRef] [PubMed]
20. Bushe, C.J.; Taylor, M.; Haukka, J. Mortality in Schizophrenia: A measurable clinical endpoint. *J. Psychopharmacol.* **2010**, *24*, 17–25. [CrossRef]
21. Pompili, M.; Amador, X.F.; Girardi, P.; Harkavy-Friedman, J.; Harrow, M.; Kaplan, K.; Montross, L.P. Suicide risk in schizophrenia: Learning from the past to change the future. *Ann. Gen. Psychiatry* **2007**, *6*, 10. [CrossRef] [PubMed]
22. Pompili, M.; Serafini, G.; Innamorati, M.; Lester, D.; Shrivastava, A.; Girardi, P.; Nordentoft, M. Suicide risk in first episode psychosis: A selective review of the current literature. *Schizophr. Res.* **2011**, *129*, 1–11. [CrossRef]
23. Cassidy, R.M.; Yang, F.; Kapczinski, F.; Passos, I.C. Risk factors for suicidality in patients with schizophrenia: A systematic review, meta-analysis, and meta-regression of 96 studies. *Schizophr. Bull.* **2018**, *44*, 787–797. [CrossRef]
24. Vrbova, K.; Prasko, J.; Ociskova, M.; Latalova, K.; Holubova, M.; Grambal, A.; Slepecky, M. Insight in schizophrenia—A double-edged sword? *Neuro. Endocrinol. Lett.* **2017**, *38*, 457–464.
25. Drake, R.; Whitaker, A.; Gates, C.; Cotton, P. Suicide among schizophrenics: A review. *Compr. Psychiatry* **1985**, *26*, 90–100. [CrossRef]
26. Togay, B.; Noyan, H.; Tasdelen, R.; Ucok, A. Clinical variables associated with suicide attempts in schizophrenia before and after the first episode. *Psychiatry Res.* **2015**, *229*, 252–256. [CrossRef]
27. Bartels, S.J.; Drake, R.E. Depressive symptoms in schizophrenia: Comprehensive differential diagnosis. *Compr. Psychiatry* **1988**, *29*, 467–483. [CrossRef]
28. Hor, K.; Taylor, M. Suicide and schizophrenia: A systematic review of rates and risk factors. *J. Psychopharmacol.* **2010**, *24*, 81–90. [CrossRef] [PubMed]
29. Strauss, J.S. Chronicity: Causes, prevention, and treatment. *Psychiatr. Ann.* **1980**, *10*, 23–29. [CrossRef]
30. Regenold, M.; Sherman, M.F.; Fenzel, M. Getting back to work: Self-efficacy as a predictor of employment outcome. *Psychiatr. Rehabil. J.* **1999**, *22*, 361. [CrossRef]
31. Hoffmann, H.; Kupper, Z.; Kunz, B. Hopelessness and its impact on rehabilitation outcome in schizophrenia–an exploratory study. *Schizophr. Res.* **2000**, *43*, 147–158. [CrossRef]
32. Cohen, L.J.; Test, M.A.; Brown, R.L. Suicide and schizophrenia: Data from a prospective community treatment study. *Am. J. Psychiatry* **1990**, *147*, 602–607.
33. Ventura, J.; Neuchterlein, K.H.; Subotnik, K.L.; Gitlin, M.J.; Sharou, J. How are self-efficacy, neurocognition, and negative symptoms related to coping responses in schizophrenia? *Schizophr. Res.* **1999**, *36*, 186–187.
34. Lysaker, P.H.; Clements, C.A.; Wright, D.E.; Evans, J.; Marks, K.A. Neurocognitive correlates of helplessness, hopelessness, and well-being in schizophrenia. *J. Nerv. Ment. Dis.* **2001**, *189*, 457–462. [CrossRef]
35. Mechanic, D.; McAlpine, D.; Rosenfield, S.; Davis, D. Effects of illness attribution and depression on the quality of life among persons with serious mental illness. *Soc. Sci. Med.* **1994**, *39*, 155–164. [CrossRef]
36. Markowitz, F.E. The effects of stigma on the psychological well-being and life satisfaction of persons with mental illness. *J. Health Soc. Behav.* **1998**, *39*, 335–347. [CrossRef]
37. Wright, E.R.; Gronfein, W.P.; Owens, T.J. Deinstitutionalization, social rejection and the self-esteem of former mental patients. *J. Health Soc. Behav.* **2000**, *41*, 68–90. [CrossRef]
38. Cotton, P.G.; Drake, R.E.; Gates, C. Critical treatment issues in suicide among schizophrenics. *Hosp. Community Psychiatry* **1985**, *36*, 534–536. [CrossRef]
39. Drake, R.E.; Gates, C.; Cotton, P.G.; Whitaker, A. Suicide among schizophrenics. Who is at risk? *J. Nerv. Ment. Dis.* **1984**, *172*, 613–617. [CrossRef]

40. Drake, R.; Cotton, P.G. Depression, hopelessness and suicide in chronic schizophrenia. *Brit. J. Psychiat.* **1986**, *148*, 554–559. [CrossRef]
41. Fenton, W.S.; McGlashan, T.H.; Victor, B.J.; Blyler, C. Symptoms, subtype, and suicidality in patients with schizophrenia spectrum disorders. *Am. J. Psychiatry.* **1997**, *154*, 199–204.
42. Nordentoft, M.; Jeppesen, P.; Abel, M.; Kassow, P.; Petersen, L.; Thorup, A.; Krarup, G.; Hemmingsen, R.; Jørgensen, P. OPUS study: Suicidal behavior, suicidal ideation and hopelessness among patients with first-episode psychosis. *Br. J. Psychiatry* **2002**, *181*, 98–106. [CrossRef]
43. Kim, C.H.; Jayathilake, K.; Meltzer, H.Y. Hopelessness, neurocognitive function, and insight in schizophrenia: Relationship to suicidal behavior. *Schizophr. Res.* **2002**, *60*, 71–80. [CrossRef]
44. Montross, L.P.; Kasckow, J.; Golshan, S.; Solorzano, E.; Lehman, D.; Zisook, S. Suicidal ideation and suicide attempts among middle-aged and older patients with schizophrenia spectrum disorders and concurrent subsyndromal depression. *J. Nerv. Ment. Dis.* **2008**, *196*, 884–890. [CrossRef]
45. Restifo, K.; Harkavy-Friedman, J.M.; Shrout, P.E. Suicidal behavior in schizophrenia. A test of the demoralization hypothesis. *J. Nerv. Ment. Dis.* **2009**, *197*, 147–153. [CrossRef] [PubMed]
46. Pompili, M.; Lester, D.; Grispini, A.; Innamorati, M.; Calandro, F.; Iliceto, P.; De Pisa, E.; Tatarelli, R.; Girardi, P. Completed suicide in schizophrenia: Evidence from a case-control study. *Psychiatry Res.* **2009**, *167*, 251–257. [CrossRef] [PubMed]
47. David Klonsky, E.; Kotov, R.; Bakst, S.; Rabinowitz, J.; Bromet, E.J. Hopelessness as a predictor of attempted suicide among first admission patients with psychosis: A 10-year cohort study. *Suicide Life-Threat. Behav.* **2012**, *42*, 1–10. [CrossRef] [PubMed]
48. Fulginiti, A.; Brekke, J.S. Escape from discrepancy: Self-esteem and quality of life as predictors of current suicidal ideation among individuals with schizophrenia. *Community Ment. Health J.* **2015**, *51*, 654–662. [CrossRef] [PubMed]
49. Tarrier, N.; Barrowclough, C.; Andrews, B.; Gregg, L. Risk of non-fatal suicide ideation and behavior in recent onset schizophrenia—The influence of clinical, social, self-esteem and demographic factors. *Soc. Psych. Psych. Epid.* **2004**, *39*, 927–937. [CrossRef]
50. Acosta, F.J.; Aguilar, E.J.; Cejas, M.R.; Gracia, R. Beliefs about illness and their relationship with hopelessness, depression, insight and suicide attempts in schizophrenia. *Psychiatr. Danub.* **2013**, *25*, 0–54.
51. Yoo, T.; Kim, S.W.; Kim, S.Y.; Lee, J.Y.; Kang, H.J.; Bae, K.Y.; Yoon, J.S. Relationship between suicidality and low self-esteem in patients with schizophrenia. *Clin. Psychopharm. Neu.* **2015**, *13*, 296. [CrossRef] [PubMed]
52. Ran, M.S.; Xiang, M.Z.; Mao, W.J.; Hou, Z.J.; Tang, M.N.; Chen, E.Y.A.; Chan, C.L.W.; Yip, P.S.F.; Conwell, Y. Characteristics of suicide attempters and nonattempters with Schizophrenia in a rural community. *Suicide Life Threat Behav.* **2005**, *35*, 694–701. [CrossRef]
53. Drake, R.J.; Pickles, A.; Bentall, R.P.; Kinderman, P.; Haddock, G.; Tarrier, N.; Lewis, S.W. The evolution of insight, paranoia and depression during early schizophrenia. *Psychol. Med.* **2004**, *34*, 285–292. [CrossRef]
54. Hasson-Ohayon, I.; Kravetz, S.; Meir, T.; Rozencwaig, S. Insight into severe mental illness, hope, and quality of life of persons with schizophrenia and schizoaffective disorders. *Psychiatry Res.* **2009**, *167*, 231–238. [CrossRef]
55. Mansouri, L.; Dowell, D.A. Perceptions of stigma among the long-term mentally ill. *Psychosoc. Rehabil. J.* **1989**, *13*, 79. [CrossRef]
56. Schulze, B.; Angermeyer, M.C. Subjective experiences of stigma. A focus group study of schizophrenic patients, their relatives and mental health professionals. *Soc. Sci. Med.* **2003**, *56*, 299–312. [CrossRef]
57. Vass, V.; Morrison, A.P.; Law, H.; Dudley, J.; Taylor, P.; Bennett, K.M.; Bentall, R.P. How stigma impacts on people with psychosis: The mediating effect of self-esteem and hopelessness on subjective recovery and psychotic experiences. *Psychiatry Res.* **2015**, *230*, 487–495. [CrossRef]
58. Birchwood, M.; Mason, R.; MacMillan, F.; Healy, J. Depression, demoralization and control over psychotic illness: A comparison of depressed and non-depressed patients with a chronic psychosis. *Psychol. Med.* **1993**, *23*, 387–395. [CrossRef] [PubMed]
59. Aguilar, E.J.; Haas, G.; Manzanera, F.J.M.; Hernández, J.; Gracia, R.; Rodado, M.J.; Keshavan, M.S. Hopelessness and first-episode psychosis: A longitudinal study. *Acta Psychiatr. Scand.* **1997**, *96*, 25–30. [CrossRef]
60. Carroll, A.; Pantelis, C.; Harvey, C. Insight and hopelessness in forensic patients with schizophrenia. *Aust. N. Z. J. Psychiatry* **2004**, *38*, 169–173. [CrossRef] [PubMed]

61. Lysaker, P.H.; Davis, L.W.; Hunter, N.L. Neurocognitive, social and clinical correlates of two domains of hopelessness in schizophrenia. *Schizophr. Res.* **2004**, *70*, 277–285. [CrossRef] [PubMed]
62. White, R.G.; McCleery, M.; Gumley, A.I.; Mulholland, C. Hopelessness in schizophrenia: The impact of symptoms and beliefs about illness. *J. Nerv. Ment. Dis.* **2007**, *195*, 968–975. [CrossRef]
63. Cavelti, M.; Kvrgic, S.; Beck, E.M.; Kossowsky, J.; Vauth, R. The role of subjective illness beliefs and attitude toward recovery within the relationship of insight and demoralization among people with schizophrenia spectrum disorders. *J. Clin. Psychol.* **2012**, *68*, 462–476. [CrossRef]
64. Cavelti, M.; Kvrgic, S.; Beck, E.M.; Rüsch, N.; Vauth, R. Self-stigma and its relationship with insight, demoralization, and clinical outcome among people with schizophrenia spectrum disorders. *Compr. Psychiatry* **2012**, *53*, 468–479. [CrossRef]
65. Boursier, S.; Jover, F.; Pringuey, D. Relevance of the concept of demoralization in schizophrenic patients. *Eur. Psychiatry* **2013**, *28*, 1. [CrossRef]
66. Wartelsteiner, F.; Mizuno, Y.; Frajo-Apor, B.; Kemmler, G.; Pardeller, S.; Sondermann, C.; Hofer, A. Quality of life in stabilized patients with schizophrenia is mainly associated with resilience and self-esteem. *Acta Psychiatr. Scand.* **2016**, *134*, 360–367. [CrossRef]
67. Touriño, R.; Acosta, F.J.; Giráldez, A.; Álvarez, J.; González, J.M.; Abelleira, C.; Benítez, N.; Baena, E.; Fernández, J.A.; Rodriguez, C.J. Suicidal risk, hopelessness and depression in patients with schizophrenia and internalized stigma. *Actas Esp. Psiquiatr.* **2018**, *46*, 33–34.
68. Upthegrove, R.; Marwaha, S.; Birchwood, M. Depression and schizophrenia: Cause, consequence, or Trans-diagnostic issue? *Schizophr. Bull.* **2017**, *43*, 240–244. [CrossRef]
69. Conley, R.R.; Ascher-Svanum, H.; Zhu, B.; Faries, D.E.; Kinon, B.J. The burden of depressive symptoms in the long-term treatment of patients with schizophrenia. *Schizophr. Res.* **2007**, *90*, 186–197. [CrossRef]
70. Gardsjord, E.S.; Romm, K.L.; Friis, S.; Barder, H.E.; Evensen, J.; Haahr, U.; Ten Velden Hegelstad, W.; Joa, I.; Johannessen, J.O.; Langeveld, J.; et al. Subjective quality of life in first-episode psychosis. A ten year follow-up study. *Schizophr. Res.* **2016**, *172*, 23–28. [CrossRef]
71. Pompili, M.; Lester, D.; Innamorati, M.; Tatarelli, R.; Girardi, P. Assessment and treatment of suicide risk in schizophrenia. *Expert Rev. Neurother.* **2008**, *8*, 51–74. [CrossRef]
72. Wetzel, R.D.; Margulies, T.; Davis, R.; Karam, E. Hopelessness, depression, and suicide intent. *J. Clin. Psychiatry* **1980**, *41*, 159–160. [CrossRef]

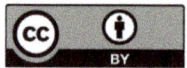

© 2019 by the authors. Licensee MDPI, Basel, Switzerland. This article is an open access article distributed under the terms and conditions of the Creative Commons Attribution (CC BY) license (http://creativecommons.org/licenses/by/4.0/).

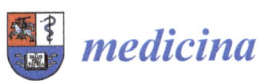

Opinion

Psychotherapy with Suicidal Patients: The Integrative Psychodynamic Approach of the Boston Suicide Study Group

Mark Schechter [1,2,*], Elsa Ronningstam [2,3], Benjamin Herbstman [2,3] and Mark J. Goldblatt [2,3]

1. North Shore Medical Center, 81 Highland Avenue, Salem, MA 01970, USA
2. Harvard Medical School, 25 Shattuck Street, Boston, MA 02115, USA; ronningstam@email.com (E.R.); bherbstman@mclean.harvard.edu (B.H.); mark_goldblatt@hms.harvard.edu (M.J.G.)
3. McLean Hospital, 115 Mill Street, Belmont, MA 02478, USA
* Correspondence: mschechter@partners.org; Tel.: +1-781-775-2724

Received: 21 March 2019; Accepted: 13 June 2019; Published: 24 June 2019

Abstract: Psychotherapy with suicidal patients is inherently challenging. Psychodynamic psychotherapy focuses attention on the patient's internal experience through the creation of a therapeutic space for an open-ended exploration of thoughts, fears, and fantasies as they emerge through interactive dialogue with an empathic therapist. The Boston Suicide Study Group (M.S., M.J.G., E.R., B.H.), has developed an integrative psychodynamic approach to psychotherapy with suicidal patients based on the authors' extensive clinical work with suicidal patients (over 100 years combined). It is fundamentally psychodynamic in nature, with an emphasis on the therapeutic alliance, unconscious and implicit relational processes, and the power of the therapeutic relationship to facilitate change in a long-term exploratory treatment. It is also integrative, however, drawing extensively on ideas and techniques described in Dialectical Behavioral Therapy (DBT), Mentalization Based Treatment (MBT), Cognitive-Behavioral Therapy (CBT), as well on developmental and social psychology research. This is not meant to be a comprehensive review of psychodynamic treatment of suicidal patients, but rather a description of an integrative approach that synthesizes clinical experience and relevant theoretical contributions from the literature that support the authors' reasoning. There are ten key aspects of this integrative psychodynamic treatment: 1. Approach to the patient in crisis; 2, instilling hope; 3. a focus on the patient's internal affective experience; 4. attention to conscious and unconscious beliefs and fantasies; 5. improving affect tolerance; 6. development of narrative identity and modification of "relational scripts"; 7. facilitation of the emergence of the patient's genuine capacities; 8. improving a sense of continuity and coherence; 9 attention to the therapeutic alliance; 10. attention to countertransference. The elements of treatment are overlapping and not meant to be sequential, but each is discussed separately as an essential aspect of the psychotherapeutic work. This integrative psychodynamic approach is a useful method for suicide prevention as it helps to instill hope, provides relational contact and engages the suicidal patient in a process that leads to positive internal change. The benefits of the psychotherapy go beyond crisis intervention, and include the potential for improved affect tolerance, more fulfilling relational experiences, emergence of previously warded off experience of genuine capacities, and a positive change in narrative identity.

Keywords: psychodynamic psychotherapy; integrative; suicide; therapeutic alliance; countertransference; hope

1. Introduction

Psychodynamic psychotherapy focuses attention on the patient's internal experience through the creation of a therapeutic space for an open-ended exploration of thoughts, fears, and fantasies as they emerge through interactive dialogue with an empathic therapist. The Boston Suicide Study Group (M.S., M.J.G., E.R., B.H.) has developed an integrative psychodynamic approach to psychotherapy with suicidal patients based on the authors' extensive clinical work with suicidal patients. It is fundamentally psychodynamic in nature, with an emphasis on the therapeutic alliance, unconscious and implicit relational processes, and the power of the therapeutic relationship to facilitate change in a long-term exploratory treatment. However, this is also an integrative approach, drawing extensively on DBT, MBT, CBT, and developmental and social psychology research. The authors have identified ten key aspects of their treatment approach: approach to the patient in crisis; instilling hope; a focus on the patient's internal affective experience; attention to conscious and unconscious beliefs and fantasies; improving affect tolerance; development of narrative identity and modification of "relational scripts"; facilitation of the emergence of the patient's genuine capacities that have been thwarted in the course of development; improving a sense of continuity and coherence; attention to the therapeutic alliance; and attention to countertransference. These elements of treatment are overlapping and are not meant to be sequential. In fact, the therapist and patient may at times be engaged in working in multiple areas fluidly and simultaneously in the course of treatment. This paper discusses each of these areas, making use of relevant literature and clinical examples to support the authors' reasoning.

Psychotherapy with suicidal patients is inherently extremely challenging. First, the therapist must accept that despite his or her best efforts there is no way to definitively control the outcome, and a patient may complete suicide. Suicidal patients are suffering terribly, and therapists are generally highly motivated to help but often lack any tools to alleviate the suffering (at least in the immediate term). Hopelessness can be particularly difficult to bear, and the therapist may feel worn down over time, beginning to accede to the patient's often stated belief that nothing can possibly be of help. In order to instill hope the therapist must have his or her own roadmap for how psychotherapy can help the patient to improve. It is our hope that this paper will help psychotherapists to understand our integrative psychodynamic approach and the ways in which it can help the patient move from suicidal despair to a life that feels worth living.

2. Background

The authors of this paper represent the Boston Suicide Study Group. We are all psychoanalysts with extensive experience in clinical work with suicidal patients (over 100 years combined) and an interest in what can be learned from integrating ideas and techniques from other psychotherapeutic approaches. We have studied and treated many psychiatric patients who have presented with suicidal ideation and plans, among them many who have made serious suicide attempts as well as some completed suicides. We have also studied the literature on psychotherapies for suicidal patients and on psychodynamic psychotherapy. This paper has been written with the intent to synthesize what we have found to be the key elements and successful treatment with suicidal patients, and to support our reasoning with relevant literature and clinical examples. It is not meant to be a comprehensive, systematic review of the literature on psychodynamic psychotherapy with suicidal patients, but rather an opportunity for us to share our integrative psychodynamic approach.

3. Elements of the Integrative Psychodynamic Approach

3.1. Approach to the Patient in Crisis

A thorough safety evaluation is essential when a patient is in an acute suicidal crisis. The therapist needs to assess the degree of imminent risk and to determine whether measures beyond psychotherapy are required to keep the patient safe (e.g., emergency department, psychiatric hospitalization, etc.). Reviews of evidence-based treatments of chronic suicidality have found that all recommend a clear frame for the treatment and a defined strategy for managing suicidal crises (i.e., a crisis plan) [1,2]. Early establishment of a treatment alliance is facilitated by the therapist's attitude of non-judgmental acceptance and validation of the patient's experience [3–5].

Patients generally enter to the clinical encounter feeling terrible about themselves, with feelings of shame, harsh self-criticism/self-attack, and a sense of hopelessness and/or failure. The therapist's empathic ability to communicate an understanding of the ways in which the patient's crisis and suicidality are understandable, given his or her situation, past experiences and current internal state, forms the foundation of the alliance. Validation helps to mitigate the experience of loneliness and aloneness, decreases self-blame and harsh self-attack, and models a hopeful attitude about the possibility that the patient can be understood and ultimately helped.

The therapist is interested in the patient's "reasons for living" [6–8], including the patient's important relationships such as family (in particularly children), to get a sense of what the patient feels there is in life to live *for*. The therapist is in a unique position to engage into a respectful dialogue with the patient, not necessarily accepting the patient's automatic defenses as the final answer. It is not uncommon, for example, for patients to say that they believe that their children "will be better off without me", as well as describe themselves as "a burden" to loved ones. With gentle confrontation and exploration, one finds that some patients actually hold more conflicted feelings and beliefs but are locked in on these explanations because it protects them from bearing the pain of their conflict and from the genuine consequences that their suicide would engender. An iterative dialogue with the therapist, in which the therapist explores and questions the patient's expressed beliefs, opens up the possibility of modification. The therapist's interest in what the patient thinks and feels about suicide and death can also be experienced as a validation, that the patient is worth the therapist's interest and engagement. The goal is not to try to control the patient's beliefs, but rather to enable the patient to experience suicidal behavior as less desirable, acceptable, and effective than the alternative of working on coping and managing distress. This can help to tip the balance away from self-destructive action [8,9].

3.2. Instilling Hope

Patients who struggle with despair and suicidality often come to the therapeutic encounter with feelings of shame, discouragement, and hopelessness. They have no "road map," of how they could possibly get from where they are feeling now to building a life worth living. The therapist can help to provide such a "road map", based on an understanding of the gains that can be achieved in the psychotherapeutic process. The patient sustains hope through the therapeutic relationship, symptom management and validation of a core identity [10], and this facilitates a gradual change in perspective on life and living.

Snyder [11] described hope as requiring both a sense of agency (sense that one has some capacity to affect positive change) and pathways (a sense of some possible routes for moving forward). The therapist holds both of these components of hope and communicates them both implicitly and directly to the patient. This helps the patient to begin to experience a sense of agency, and to have some glimmer of how he or she can survive the current feelings and go on to have a life worth living. Helping to sustain the therapist's hope is the data that suicidal behavior is often a transient phenomenon. Studies have found that the vast majority of people who survive even the most severe suicide attempts actually do not go on to kill themselves [12,13]. Psychotherapy has been found to reduce the risk of recurrent suicide attempts and self-injury [14].

Psychotherapy can help support the patient who is engaging in an internal process that can gradually lead to a changed perspective and greater hope for the future. One aspect of this process is a genuine acceptance of the actual conditions that precipitated the suicidal crisis. This is especially important for patients who have faced drastic changes in life (e.g., losses, humiliations, etc.), or are coming to a realization that life is not going to turn out as expected or envisioned. Related to this is a person's ability to tolerate and accept loss, sadness, and disappointment. This involves a process of grief and mourning for what one had and will never have again, and/or what could have been but will not be. It requires engagement of the patient's self-reflective capacity, which is facilitated in psychotherapy by validation of the patient's pain, modeling reflection, affective engagement and modulation of the patient's harsh self-criticism/self-attack and feelings of failure.

Over time, the therapist can support the patient in moving from a fixation on what is ideal, to recognizing the possibility of what can be good enough. Early in the process, the "good enough" is often devalued and depicted as not worth living for, but with ongoing reflection, mourning, and support, the patient can learn that it is possible to find meaning and even joy in life with goals and expectations that have shifted in line with what is possible. This includes a re-engagement in relationships and a greater sense of belonging. At the same time, mobilization of the patient's sense of agency and instilling of hope for the future can lead to actions on the patient's part that can have a positive impact on relationships and circumstances. This can create a positive feedback loop that can lead to actual achievements beyond what the patient could have envisioned in a prior state of hopelessness.

3.3. Focus on Internal Experience and Affect

A distinguishing aspect of psychodynamic psychotherapy is the close attention to the patient's internal experience. Shneidman eloquently described suicide as 'a combined movement toward cessation and away from intolerable, unendurable, unacceptable anguish' ([15], p. 6). Multiple other terms have been used in the literature to describe this affective state by many differing theoretical orientations, trying to capture essentially the same experience: It has been variously referred to as "desperation" [16], "mental pain" [17], "psychache" [18], "emotional dysregulation" [3], and "annihilation anxiety" [19]. Hendin et al. [16] found that therapists reported a higher number of intense, agonizing affective states in patients who completed suicide in the course of psychotherapy, as compared with a severely depressed, non-suicidal comparison group. The most frequently cited affect was desperation, defined as a state of anguish accompanied by an urgent need for relief. More recently, Galynker [20] has focused on "entrapment", an emotional experience of desperation with no perceived way out.

The state of "aloneness" has been described as an unbearable experience that makes people feel desperate and puts them at risk for suicidal behavior [21,22]. Joiner and colleagues have studied a closely related experience, that of "thwarted belongingness", and found it to be a key factor in making completion of suicide possible [23,24]. Maltsberger [22] described aloneness as "an experience beyond hope . . . . This anxiety is the anxiety of annihilation—panic and terror. People will do anything to escape from this experience" (p. 50). The experience can feel timeless, as though once it has started it will continue for every, which adds to the sense of desperation. Aloneness is qualitatively different from loneliness, which is contingent and time limited. It is the loss of capacity to *experience* the closeness and caring of others, even if they are present and available.

In the face of an unrelenting, unbearable affective experience, cognition changes in a way that makes rational problem solving much more difficult. Baumeister [25] described the suicidal patient as moving into a state of cognitive "deconstruction" (pp. 92–93), characterized by rigidity, increasingly concrete thinking. a narrowing of sense of time to the present and an exclusive focus on immediate goals, and a lack of integration and meaning. Linehan [3] has observed that in states of severe emotional dysregulation, patients often lose certain capacities that they have in a calmer state of mind. Thinking becomes much more concrete and constricted; when the patient sees no alternative, no endpoint or escape, the risk of suicidal behavior is increased. Maltsberger [26] described the traumatic state of disintegration that accompanies a suicidal state.

An unbearable affective experience is distinct from depression. For vulnerable patients, it can come on suddenly, in response to a stressor, at times without the patient making the connection between stress and response. It can also be relieved transiently if the patient is suddenly provided a respite, such as by psychiatric hospitalization. The relief, however, can be suddenly and overwhelmingly reversed when the patient is re-exposed to overwhelming stressors at discharge, which is probably a major factor in the high rate of post-discharge suicide [27]. Ideally, psychotherapeutic efforts in the hospital can be targeted toward helping the patient to anticipate and problem-solve for upcoming crises, and to develop a usable and well-practiced crisis plan. It is important for the therapist to be aware that the immediate period post-discharge is very high risk for the patient, and to intervene accordingly.

3.4. Attention to Patients Conscious and Unconscious Beliefs and Fantasies

Psychodynamic psychotherapy provides an opportunity to explore the patient's conscious and unconscious beliefs and fantasies about suicide. These fantasies are often not rational and in contradiction with the patient's known reality. The idea of suicide can have very different meanings and can be facilitated or mitigated by different sets of fantasies. Some may be conscious, and others may be out of their awareness. These beliefs and fantasies can be wide ranging, and at times in contradiction with each other and/or with reality. Some patients believe they deserve punishment; others long for a fantasized reunion with lost parents or a loved one; some have a fantasy that they will get to "see" the reaction of others to the suicide, and even that they will experience pleasure in doing so, even while knowing rationally that this is not the case; some experience their body as hateful and want to destroy it, perhaps because it is identified with a past abuser (see [28]).

The patient's fantasies about suicide and death can influence the likelihood of suicidal action. Articulating and exploring these fantasies enables a therapeutic dialogue which gives the therapist the opportunity to respectfully challenge certain automatic assumptions. For example, perhaps the mother who states the belief that her child would be better off without her, is in fact able and willing to consider the possibility that she might be misreading the situation because of her depression and despair. A man who is experiencing aloneness and has a fantasy of rejoining his deceased wife in heaven may be willing to consider the possibility that suicide might *not* mean a blissful reunion, and that there are other consequences that he is not letting himself think through. The therapist's interest in exploring the patient's fantasies demonstrates his or her wish to get a full understanding of the patient's experience, and in this way may bolster the patient's sense that he or she matters. It also provides an opportunity for gradual modification of these beliefs in the context of an iterative dialogue over time.

Some suicidal contemplation and fantasy can be "self-sustaining". Rather than facilitating action, these thoughts can help to calm people down and help them regulate affect in a way that helps preclude the need to act on suicide [29]. These are often patients for whom the idea that they could complete suicide has served as a psychological "out" which gives them a feeling of *potential* escape from their distress; as long as they hold onto suicide as an option, they do not need to act. This kind of suicidal contemplation is "a self-soothing measure and an aid to narcissistic cohesion" (p. 612). Patients often do not understand this distinction and may be very troubled by their suicidal thoughts even as it serves an important function for them. The therapist can reassure the patient about the role of suicidal fantasy, and that thoughts do not equate with action. In fact, in the general population the ratio of those who harbor suicidal thoughts to those who kill themselves is over 200:1 [30].

3.5. Improving Affect Tolerance

Increasing affect tolerance is central to psychotherapy with patients with emotional dysregulation. Affect tolerance might roughly be defined as increasing one's capacity to think in the presence of strong emotions, and to bear feelings without having to suppress, dissociate, or act impulsively. In Dialectical Behavior Therapy (DBT), emotion regulation and distress tolerance skills are targeted to increase affect tolerance [3]. The therapist may integrate teaching the patient these skills in a psychodynamic treatment frame.

Perhaps unique to psychodynamic therapy is the opportunity to work with the patient on unconscious fears and avoidances that have a profound effect on the patient's sense of self, transferences, core beliefs, and relationships. The patient brings his or her sense of shame, humiliation, and feelings of despair to the treatment, often unconsciously fearing negative reaction on the part of the therapist that comes from a template of past relationships. Ideally with validation and support, these feelings can gradually extinguish, giving the patient more flexibility and choice. People are unaware of automatic avoidance defenses and are highly motivated to continue to use them to ward off anxiety provoking and conflictual thoughts and feelings. This keeps such material out of consciousness, and unavailable to be worked on in therapy. When the therapist gently notices avoidant defenses (e.g., "when I said that, I noticed you averted your eyes and started to change the subject ... what was going on there?"), it offers the patient an opportunity to consider what he or she is warding off. At times, the therapist may use explicit exposure techniques (e.g., "can you try saying that again while looking me in the eye, and just sit with what you are feeling?") in order to facilitate the patient's exposure to underlying uncomfortable feelings that are being warded off. With ongoing therapy, the need for these automatic avoidant defenses gradually begins to lessen. The extinguishing of shame, fear, expectancies of harsh attacks/blame, etc., allows for greater tolerance of affect, increasing the patient's flexibility and freedom of expression. This work is closely related to work on narrative identity (described below), with the working through of the patient's "relational scripts" that have led to recurrent experiences that sustain negative ideas/beliefs/conclusions about self.

3.6. Narrative Identity and "Relational Scripts"

The development of personal "narratives" has been found to be critical to the establishment and ongoing development of identity [31–37] People tell themselves stories to link experiences, make meaning from events, establish a sense of continuity of experience, and articulate ways in which they have changed [38]. In this way, people develop a "life story," described as "an internalized and evolving narrative of the self that selectively reconstructs the past and anticipates the future in such a way as to provide a life with an overall sense of coherence and purpose" ([36], p. 1372). The personal narratives of the depressed or suicidal patient's self-narrative are generally harshly self-critical and negative (e.g., "Everything I try to do fails I never get things right"). Galynker described the "suicidal narrative" as telling the story of "a present that is so intolerable that the future becomes unimaginable" ([20], p. 31).

Personal narratives are actually co-constructed, with the listener influencing whether and how the story is told, and meanings that can be derived from it [33,39,40]. Sharing one's personal stories with others helps to make meaning from experiences, and to try out ways of understanding oneself. Psychodynamic psychotherapy provides an opportunity for the patient to engage with a new "listener," an active participant who engages in the development of the patient's narrative [37]. The therapist notices and takes up the harsh self-criticism and self-attack embedded in the patient's story, and in so doing begins a process of modification.

Patients often begin treatment with a narrative that does not "connect the dots" between past experience and current despair. A patient might tell a story of severe neglect and/or abuse that clearly would lead to problems with self-esteem and trust but not make this connection. Together, therapist and patient engage in an iterative dialogue in which the patient's narrative is reworked and co-constructed. Not all patients come into treatment with the capacity to share a coherent narrative, particularly in the context of neglectful and abusive early experiences. Problems may occur at the "pre-narrative" and "proto-narrative" levels at which mental images are generated and linked to emotions, which eventually become the building blocks for higher level, verbal, narrative construction [41]. Early trauma and neglect can lead to a lack of emotional marking of mental images and an inability to recruit these images into meaningful sequences that integrate cognition and emotion. As a result, narratives are disorganized, impoverished, and sometimes frankly incoherent, and "the therapist finds it difficult to comprehend the patient's mental state" (p. 236). This leads to problems with self-cohesion and emotion regulation. Psychotherapy can help the patient to link emotions, mental images narrative fragments, and behavior with a goal of increasing self-coherence.

Early attachment and caregiver experiences form the foundation for development of Identity and sense of self in relation to others. The infant/child requires recognition and marking of mental and emotional states in order to develop their own capacity to recognize, label, and ultimately modulate emotions [42–44]. This is foundational for the development of mentalization, the ability to appreciate and reflect on the mental states of others. The child who is not recognized and "kept in mind" is bound to have difficulties in self-recognition at multiple levels, and to be more vulnerable to states of disorganization, overwhelming affect, and experiences of aloneness. The individual develops the "inner working models" [45] or "implicit relational scripts" [46–48] from the relational experiences with early caregivers. These models define how one experiences oneself, and therefore how one acts, in relation to others. "These are the automatic procedural relationship rules that one lives by, generally without awareness: "This is how people experience me; this is how I am valued, or not valued, by others; this is how I tend to be treated; this is how my relationships go; this is what happens when I make my wishes and needs known; this is who I am" ([37], p. 29)."

Implicit beliefs about self and relational patterns tend to be tenacious and resistant to change. Studies in social psychology have found that people tend to "self-verify," seeking and selectively attending to feedback that confirms and reinforces the way that they already see themselves [49–51]. From an analytic perspective, Wachtel [52] described how people actively (although non-consciously) elicit confirmation of their self-concept by acting in ways that tend to evoke confirmatory responses; thus, the patient receives ongoing reinforcement that sustains his or her self-concept, even if that experience is terribly painful. The therapist engages the patient and disrupts the patient's nonconscious relational scripts by behaving differently than was unconsciously expected, thus offering the possibility that the therapeutic relationship has the potential to facilitate change. The therapist also attends to the myriad of relational experiences that continue to reinforce and sustain the patient's self-beliefs and behaviors. This means actively helping the patient to create new relational experiences that disrupt the repetitive elicitation of social feedback that confirms and sustains the patient's maladaptive beliefs about self.

The therapist's activity may include what are traditionally thought of as cognitive-behavioral strategies (e.g., problem-solving, modeling alternative ways of relating, exposure, role playing) to help the patient navigate difficult relational situations with the best possible chance to have positive and 'script disrupting' experiences. This is an iterative process, with repeated discrepant experiences with the therapist and with others gradually modifying the underlying dysfunctional relational scripts. It is especially critical in the psychotherapy of those who are vulnerable to suicidal states, for whom the repeated nonconscious evocation of confirmatory negative interpersonal experiences can quickly lead to turmoil and despair, making suicidal behavior more likely. This will be discussed further in the discussion below about the therapeutic alliance.

3.7. The Emergence and Recognition of the Patient's Genuine Capacities

The emerging recognition and appreciation of one's genuine capacities is a developmental process that can be derailed through trauma or other negative developmental experiences [37,53]. Loewald [54] described the importance of the analyst in this regard, holding and communicating a vision of the patient as who he or she is, as well as the "more" that he or she can come to be. Patients who are vulnerable to suicidal states often have anxiety associated with experiencing themselves positively, with harsh self-attack and automatic avoidant defenses that keep them from fully taking in positive relational and other experiences. The therapist, by noticing this nonconscious avoidance, calls attention to and thereby disrupts these defenses in a way that gives the patient an opportunity to bear the anxiety and conflict associated with experiencing oneself more fully. At times, this can mean integrating more formal exposure into the treatment (e.g., "I noticed when you talked about the 'A' that you got in class, you looked away and started to mumble … What were you feeling? Maybe you can say it again but try to look right at me and use a strong voice. Let's see if you can sit with the feelings that this brings up."). Over time, the anxiety begins to diminish, and the patient gradually begins to feel more comfortable with a more complete experience of himself or herself. This creates a positive feedback loop as the patient also begins to act in a way that is consistent with his or her emerging identity and thus is more likely to elicit, and attend to, confirmatory feedback (53), which has been described as a renegotiation of identity [50].

3.8. Continuity and Coherence

Continuity is the sense of being the same person with linked experiences over time; coherence has to do with linking experiences, roles and beliefs as part of an integrated whole [35]. Patients with Borderline Personality Disorder (BPD) have been described as being vulnerable to a sudden loss of continuity—the loss of evocative memory—that leaves them unable to evoke soothing introjects and acutely vulnerable to experiences of aloneness and suicidal desperation [21]. Maltsberger [27] envisioned the "descent into suicide" as an overwhelming, unbearable flooding of negative affect that leads to a breakup of self-cohesion, to which those who do not have a strong base of continuity of self are particularly vulnerable.

Severe distress becomes unbearable when one loses the capacity to experience connection with others, a state of excruciating aloneness. This becomes even more dire "with the loss of a continuous thread of being that mitigates the sense that now is all there is, that pain will be forever, that there is no hope of moving forward because there is no forward, and that suicide might be the only option" ([37], p. 34). Recurrent affective dysregulation, mood changes and psychotic experiences can themselves be experienced as traumatic and are disruptive to developing and sustaining continuity and coherence [19].

What this means is that the therapist should consider a sense of continuity and coherence a treatment goal rather than an expectation [37]. The therapist, at times, may need to painstakingly help the patient link experiences with each other, reminding the patient that aspects of the past continue to influence the present, and even helping the patient to link dissociated experiences day-to-day. Some patients are vulnerable to feeling suddenly disconnected, alone and desperate, without any sense that something may have happened to cause their change in mental state, and the timeless sense that they will never feel better again. At these moments, the therapist may help the patient through these experiences by inter-session contact of some kind (e.g., phone, email, voice mail), and also by helping the patient to connect feelings with experiences to begin to understand the transient vulnerability to these dissociated states.

3.9. Attention to the Therapeutic Alliance

Building and maintaining a strong therapeutic alliance is a cornerstone of psychotherapy with suicidal patients, but it is fraught with significant challenges (see [55,56]). Psychotherapy often involves strong transference–countertransference reactions to which both patient and therapist contribute. Patients often come to the encounter with intense affects, and negative relational expectations. Negative therapeutic reactions and treatment crises are common, and often inculcate a fear of catastrophic consequences. Dealing with these inherent difficulties is a challenge for both patient and therapist and is critical to the success of the therapy [57–59].

A related challenge for the therapist is the need to move flexibly between empathic listening and an ongoing suicide risk assessment [55,56]. The therapist shifts between creating a psychotherapeutic space and observing the patient objectively. When there is a change in the patient's emotional state or degree of relatedness, the therapist begins an assessment of the patient's safety, the strength of the alliance, and whether there is a need for other safety interventions. Anxiety about the patient's safety can paradoxically take the therapist away from a stance of empathic attunement.

Suicidal patients generally have a harshly self-critical internal narrative, and an underlying expectation of negative interpersonal experiences that confirm their bad sense of self. In this context, the therapist needs to be actively affirmative and validating in order to achieve "functional neutrality" [60]. One issue on which psychodynamics differ is how to conceptualize and to manage the patient's aggression and negative transference. Transference Focused Psychotherapy (TFP), for example, prioritizes interpreting aggressive, split off, unintegrated parts, and considers this an essential element even early in the course of treatment [61]. Our approach prioritizes attunement to the patient's internal experience (as experienced by the patient), which we see as essential to strengthening the alliance and helping the patient with the experience of aloneness. We conceptualize aggression as most often a secondary response to the patient's internal state of desperation. A metaphor that we find helpful is that of a person who is drowning, unable to breathe, and who desperately grasps for a life raft, pushing past and inadvertently injuring another person. One could take up the aggression as primary, but we do not feel that this is closest to the patient's experience, for whom the lashing out came from a desperate effort to breathe and to stay alive. This is very much akin to the suicidal patient's desperate experience of aloneness, abandonment, and other unbearable emotional experiences, which leads to an urgent need for relief/escape. We do not ignore aggression and take it up as needed to preserve the treatment and the frame. However, in our view, interpreting the negative transference, especially for early in treatment, can be experienced as distant and critical, which is antithetical to our goal of the early attunement and validation. In this way, we are very much aligned with the approach in Mentalization Based Therapy (MBT), with an emphasis on validation of the patient's transference feeling, avoiding genetic interpretations that might be experienced as distancing and invalidating, exploring the transference, attending closely to the therapist's contribution to the patient's transference experience, and collaborative exploration [62].

The strength of the therapeutic alliance, including rupture and successful repair of the alliance, is a critical factor in the success of any psychotherapy (see [56–58]). In working with emotionally dysregulated patients, ruptures in the alliance can be particularly abrupt and severe—sometimes in response to something that occurs in the therapy, sometimes related to external stressors—with a risk of affective turmoil and potential for suicidal behavior. These ruptures can be extremely difficult for the therapist as well as for the patient, but if they can be repaired, they offer an opportunity for implicit relational learning and growth. In this context:

> ... the patient has the chance to discover experientially that an old relational pattern does not have to be repeated, and that the therapeutic relationship holds the promise of trying out, practicing and even solidifying something new. The patient also has the chance to learn that the therapist, and the relationship, can survive the intensity of the patient's sudden withdrawal or affective storm. These moments are essential in gradually building trust, in strengthening the emotional bond between patient and therapist and in holding out the hope that the relationship might actually be of help ([56], p. 319).

In this reworking of the script, the patient has an opportunity to experience the therapist as caring, and himself or herself as being worthy of being cared about. Working through ruptures often requires that the patient experience something different from the therapist, in some way above and beyond what the patient expected. This might be in the form of a self-disclosure (e.g., the therapist might acknowledge an unempathetic reaction, and share that something about what the patient had said reminded him or her of a troubling experience), an action (e.g., having the patient stay a few minutes beyond the hour because of the importance of the patient's association), or some other spontaneous and genuine way of relating to the patient.

Stern et al. [46] described the therapeutic importance of "moments of meeting," in which "the therapist must use a specific aspect of his or her individuality that carries a personal signature. The two are meeting as persons relatively unhidden by their usual therapeutic roles, for that moment" (p. 913). Linehan [4] used the term "radical genuineness" to capture the same experience. Hoffman [63], writing about psychoanalysis, captured the implicit meaning in the therapist's doing something that is experienced as different in response to the patient's need:

> When the patient senses that the analyst, in becoming more personally expressive and involved, is departing from an internalized convention of some kind, the patient has reason to feel recognized in a special way, the deviation, whatever its content and whatever the nature of the pressure from the patient, may reflect an emotional engagement on the analyst's part that is responsive in a unique way to this particular patient ... there is something about the deviation itself, regardless of content, that has therapeutic potential (pp. 187–193).

Similarly, the patient may require measures that go beyond the traditional frame of the psychotherapy session to maintain or regain an empathic connection [64]. Interventions such as between session contact, offering additional sessions, and intermittent telephone, email or text support can help the patient cope with affective intensity when in crisis. These actions may also have internal meaning for the patient, serving to enhance internalization of the therapist as a positive introject and strengthen the therapeutic alliance [56]. Thoughtful flexibility regarding the treatment frame can be experienced as validating by the patient (i.e., the therapist cares enough to be flexible and is willing to prioritize the patient's perceived needs) and often helps to strengthen and solidify the therapeutic alliance. In cases of severe personality disorders such as antisocial and severely narcissistic personality disorders, it may at times be beneficial to set and adhere to a more rigid frame (such as that advocated in TFP) [61]. On the other hand, a strict requirement for adherence to a set frame may evoke feelings of being controlled and entrapped, and in some circumstances can hinder the development of the alliance. In our view, it is important that the patient experiences agency in the treatment and feels that the therapist is listening and taking seriously his or her concerns, with some degree of flexibility. This is best accomplished through a sensitive and proactive collaborative negotiation with the patient around frame issues, with attention to the patient's wishes and perceived needs, therapeutic goals, and the therapist's personal limits.

Patients who have experienced traumatic affective experiences (not just overt trauma and neglect, but also truly overwhelming and unbearable affective experiences and psychotic states) are vulnerable to an erosion of the capacity to fully engage with sustaining relationships [19]. In this context, it can be too hard for the patient to sustain hope, and too easy to begin to give up on the ties to loved ones that are life-sustaining. If the patient can experience the therapist's genuine affective involvement—at both a cognitive and implicit relational level—this can be the first step to regaining some hope for change. The therapist's effort at repair, experienced as genuine and emotionally resonant by the patient, "is inviting the patient to hang on, to turn towards the relationship instead of away from it and to use the therapist's help to find ways to cope without resorting to suicide" ([56], p. 320).

3.10. Attention to Countertransference

Psychotherapy with suicidal patients is inherently extremely challenging. First, the therapist must accept that despite his or her best efforts there is no way to definitively control the outcome, and a patient may complete suicide. The lack of control about a potentially catastrophic outcome for which the therapist may feel blamed engenders anxiety, fear, and other emotions that are inescapable. In addition, repeatedly sitting with a patient who is in terrible emotional pain, without the means to provide relief, is a very difficult emotional task for the therapist.

Hopelessness can be particularly difficult to bear, and the therapist may feel worn down over time, beginning to accede to the patient's often stated belief that nothing can possibly be of help [55]. In most cases, this is a "countertransference hopelessness" which can unconsciously be communicated to the patient in verbal interaction and also in non-verbal cues. This then invites feelings of aloneness and abandonment in the patient, increasing hopelessness. The therapist can use his or her own reflective capacity, internal sustaining resources, knowledge about psychotherapeutic potential for change, and clinical experience to balance these reactions to the patient and to maintain hope. Consultation with a colleague or supervisor or a colleague can be effective in helping the therapist to regain balance and re-engage with the patient.

Suicidal patients are suffering terribly, and therapists are highly motivated to help, but often lack any tools to alleviate the suffering (at least in the immediate term). This can activate multiple affects in the therapist and trigger unconscious defense mechanisms. The therapist may feel suddenly anxious, overwhelmed, frustrated, and hopeless. The therapist's automatic defenses against such feelings may include avoidance of affect; exclusive focus on symptoms rather than feelings; efforts to control the patient's behavior, or an opposite lack of engagement in the patient's decision-making; and denial about the seriousness of the patient's distress. In their classic paper, Maltsberger and Buie [65] discuss the "countertransference hate" that can arise in the therapist. They describe two components: "malice" which is a more overt experience leading to expression of irritation or anger towards the patient, and the even more concerning "aversion", which represents unconscious emotional withdrawal. It is the latter, aversion, that is most scary in terms of increasing potential suicide risk, as patients tend to be exquisitely attuned to the therapist's emotional state and level of engagement. Unconscious withdrawal by the therapist may be experienced with an increase in aloneness and a sense of abandonment, which can put the patient at risk for despair and suicidal behavior. Again, discussion with colleagues and formal consultation can be extremely helpful for the therapist to get out of the intensity of the dyad and to explore his or her feelings about the patient and the treatment.

4. Conclusions

In this paper, the Boston Suicide Study Group has presented a theoretical and clinical approach to psychotherapy with suicidal patients. It is fundamentally a psychodynamic treatment, with an emphasis on the therapeutic alliance, unconscious and implicit relational processes, and the power of the therapeutic relationship to facilitate change in a long-term exploratory treatment. It is also integrative, incorporating ideas from DBT, MBT, and CBT, developmental and social psychology in a psychodynamic frame. There are ten key aspects of this integrative psychodynamic treatment: 1. approach to the patient in crisis; 2, instilling hope; 3. a focus on the patient's internal affective experience; 4. attention to conscious and unconscious beliefs and fantasies; 5. improving affect tolerance; 6. development of narrative identity and modification of "relational scripts"; 7. facilitation of the emergence of the patient's genuine capacities; 8. improving a sense of continuity and coherence; 9 attention to the therapeutic alliance; 10. attention to countertransference. These elements of treatment are overlapping and are not meant to be sequential, but they provide a "road map" of the various ways in which this psychotherapy facilitates a patient's move from despair and suicidality to a more satisfying relational experience with others.

Engagement with an empathic therapist provides a secure environment for exploration of the suicidal patient's internal subjective experience. The therapist helps to instill hope by bearing the patient's pain while helping the patient to discover and mobilize a sense of agency, mourn what truly is not possible, re-engage in relationships, and begin to envision a life that is worth living. The therapist notices and disrupts the patient's non-conscious defenses, leading to exposure to previously warded off feelings and greater affect tolerance. In listening to and engaging in the patient's narrative, the therapist helps to co-construct a new narrative that is more empathic and less self-attacking, renegotiating narrative identity in a more realistic and positive way. The therapist facilitates the gradual emergence of the patient's genuine capacities, modulating self-attack and disrupting avoidant defenses, and providing the patient an opportunity to bear the anxiety and conflict associated with experiencing oneself more fully. Great attention is paid to the therapeutic alliance and the therapist's countertransference.

The therapist engages with and disrupts the patient's nonconscious relational scripts by behaving differently than unconsciously expected, thus offering the possibility that the therapeutic relationship has the potential to facilitate change. At the same time, the therapist actively supports the patient in creating new relational experiences that begin to elicit feedback that is discrepant with maladaptive core beliefs about self. Ruptures in the therapeutic alliance can be extremely painful, but repair of the alliance offers a further opportunity for implicit relational learning and growth.

Author Contributions: Writing—original draft, M.S.; Writing—review and editing, E.R., B.H. and M.G.

Funding: This research received no external funding.

Acknowledgments: The authors wish to acknowledge John T. (Terry) Maltsberger, who was a mentor to all of us and the leader of the Boston Suicide Study Group. While Terry was not with us for the preparation of this manuscript, he was ever present in our hearts and minds. We are forever grateful for his wisdom and friendship.

Conflicts of Interest: The authors declare no conflict of interest.

References

1. Weinberg, I.; Ronningstam, E.; Goldblatt, M.J.; Schechter, M.; Wheelis, J.; Maltsberger, J.T. Strategies in Treatment of Suicidality: Identification of Common and Treatment-Specific Interventions in Empirically Supported Treatment Manuals. *J. Clin. Psychiatry* **2010**, *71*, 699–706. [CrossRef] [PubMed]
2. Sledge, W.; Plakun, E.M.; Bauer, S.; Brodsky, B.; Caligor, E.; Clemens, N.A.; Deen, S.; Kay, J.; Lazar, S.; Mellman, L.A.; et al. Psychotherapy for suicidal patients with borderline personality disorder: An expert consensus review of common factors across five therapies. *Bord. Personal. Disord. Emot. Dysregul.* **2014**, *1*, 16. [CrossRef] [PubMed]
3. Linehan, M. *Cognitive-Behavioral Treatment of Borderline Personality Disorder*; Diagnosis and Treatment of Mental Disorders; Guilford Press: New York, NY, USA, 1993; ISBN 978-0-89862-183-9.
4. Linehan, M.M. Validation and psychotherapy. In *Empathy Reconsidered: New Directions in Psychotherapy*; Bohart, A.C., Greenberg, L.S., Eds.; American Psychological Association: Washington, DC, USA, 1997; pp. 353–392. ISBN 978-1-55798-410-4.
5. Schechter, M. The Patient's Experience of Validation in Psychoanalytic Treatment. *J. Am. Psychoanal. Assoc.* **2007**, *55*, 105–130. [CrossRef] [PubMed]
6. Linehan, M.M.; Goodstein, J.L.; Nielsen, S.L.; Chiles, J.A. Reasons for staying alive when you are thinking of killing yourself: The reasons for living inventory. *J. Consult. Clin. Psychol.* **1983**, *51*, 276–286. [CrossRef] [PubMed]
7. Strosahl, K.; Chiles, J.A.; Linehan, M. Prediction of suicide intent in hospitalized parasuicides: Reasons for living, hopelessness, and depression. *Compr. Psychiatry* **1992**, *33*, 366–373. [CrossRef]
8. Malone, K.M.; Oquendo, M.A.; Haas, G.L.; Ellis, S.P.; Li, S.; Mann, J.J. Protective Factors Against Suicidal Acts in Major Depression: Reasons for Living. *Am. J. Psychiatry* **2000**, *157*, 1084–1088. [CrossRef]
9. Chiles, J.A.; Strosahl, K.D.; McMurtray, L.; Linehan, M.M. Modeling effects on suicidal behavior. *J. Nerv. Ment. Dis.* **1985**, *173*, 477–481. [CrossRef]
10. Goldblatt, M.J. The psychodynamics of hope in suicidal despair. *Scand. Psychoanal. Rev.* **2017**, *40*, 54–62. [CrossRef]
11. Snyder, C.R. TARGET ARTICLE: Hope Theory: Rainbows in the Mind. *Psychol. Inq.* **2002**, *13*, 249–275. [CrossRef]
12. Seiden, R.H. Where are they now? A follow-up study of suicide attempters from the Golden Gate Bridge. *Suicide Life Threat. Behav.* **1978**, *8*, 203–216.
13. Suominen, K.; Isometsä, E.; Suokas, J.; Haukka, J.; Achte, K.; Lönnqvist, J. Completed Suicide After a Suicide Attempt: A 37-Year Follow-Up Study. *Am. J. Psychiatry* **2004**, *161*, 562–563. [CrossRef] [PubMed]
14. Calati, R.; Courtet, P. Is psychotherapy effective for reducing suicide attempt and non-suicidal self-injury rates? Meta-analysis and meta-regression of literature data. *J. Psychiatr. Res.* **2016**, *79*, 8–20. [CrossRef] [PubMed]
15. Shneidman, E. What do suicides have in common? Summary of the psychological approach. In *Suicide: Guidelines for Assessment, Management, and Treatment*; Bongar, B.M., Ed.; Oxford University Press: New York, NY, USA, 1992; pp. 3–15. ISBN 978-0-19-506846-7.
16. Hendin, H.; Maltsberger, J.T.; Haas, A.P.; Szanto, K.; Rabinowicz, H. Desperation and Other Affective States in Suicidal Patients. *Suicide Life Threat. Behav.* **2004**, *34*, 386–394. [CrossRef] [PubMed]
17. Orbach, I.; Mikulincer, M.; Gilboa-Schechtman, E.; Sirota, P. Mental Pain and Its Relationship to Suicidality and Life Meaning. *Suicide Life Threat. Behav.* **2003**, *33*, 231–241. [CrossRef] [PubMed]
18. Shneidman, E.S. Commentary: Suicide as Psychache. *J. Nerv. Ment. Dis.* **1993**, *181*, 145–147. [CrossRef]
19. Maltsberger, J.T.; Goldblatt, M.J.; Ronningstam, E.; Weinberg, I.; Schechter, M. Traumatic Subjective Experiences Invite Suicide. *J. Am. Acad. Psychoanal. Dyn. Psychiatry* **2011**, *39*, 671–693. [CrossRef] [PubMed]
20. Galynker, I.I. *The Suicidal Crisis: Clinical Guide to the Assessment of Imminent Suicide Risk*; Oxford University Press: New York, NY, USA, 2018; ISBN 978-0-19-026085-9.
21. Adler, G.; Buie, D.H. Aloneness and borderline psychopathology: The possible relevance of child development issues. *Int. J. Psychoanal.* **1979**, *60*, 83–96. [PubMed]
22. Maltsberger, J.T. Suicide Danger: Clinical Estimation and Decision. *Suicide Life Threat. Behav.* **1988**, *18*, 47–54. [CrossRef] [PubMed]

23. Joiner, T.E. *Why People Die by Suicide*; Harvard University Press: Cambridge, MA, USA, 2005; ISBN 978-0-674-01901-0.
24. Van Orden, K.A.; Witte, T.K.; Cukrowicz, K.C.; Braithwaite, S.R.; Selby, E.A.; Joiner, T.E. The interpersonal theory of suicide. *Psychol. Rev.* **2010**, *117*, 575–600. [CrossRef]
25. Baumeister, R.F. Suicide as escape from self. *Psychol. Rev.* **1990**, *97*, 90–113. [CrossRef]
26. Maltsberger, J.T. The descent into suicide. *Int. J. Psychoanal.* **2004**, *85*, 653–668. [CrossRef] [PubMed]
27. Schechter, M.; Goldblatt, M.J.; Ronningstam, E.; Herbstman, B.; Maltsberger, J.T. Postdischarge suicide: A psychodynamic understanding of subjective experience and its importance in suicide prevention. *Bull. Menn. Clin.* **2016**, *80*, 80–96. [CrossRef] [PubMed]
28. Maltsberger, J.T.; Buie, D.H. The devices of suicide. Revenge, riddance, and rebirth. *Int. Rev. Psychoanal.* **1980**, *7*, 61–72.
29. Maltsberger, J.T.; Ronningstam, E.; Weinberg, I.; Schechter, M.; Goldblatt, M.J. Suicide fantasy as a life-sustaining recourse. *J. Am. Acad Psychoanal. Dyn. Psychiatry* **2010**, *38*, 611–623. [CrossRef] [PubMed]
30. Baldessarini, R.J. *Suicide Risks: Rates & Predictors in Major Mood Disorders and Post-Discharge*; McLean Hospital Grand Rounds: Belmont, MA, USA, 2019.
31. McAdams, D.P. Personality, Modernity, and the Storied Self: A Contemporary Framework for Studying Persons. *Psychol. Inq.* **1996**, *7*, 295–321. [CrossRef]
32. McAdams, D.P. The psychology of life stories. *Rev. Gen. Psychol.* **2001**, *5*, 100–122. [CrossRef]
33. Thorne, A. Personal memory telling and personality development. *Pers. Soc. Psychol. Rev.* **2000**, *4*, 45–56. [CrossRef]
34. Pasupathi, M. The social construction of the personal past and its implications for adult development. *Psychol. Bull.* **2001**, *127*, 651–672. [CrossRef]
35. Pasupathi, M. Identity: Commentary: Identity Development: Dialogue Between Normative and Pathological Developmental Approaches. *J. Personal. Disord.* **2014**, *28*, 113–120. [CrossRef]
36. McAdams, D.P.; Bauer, J.J.; Sakaeda, A.R.; Anyidoho, N.A.; Machado, M.A.; Magrino-Failla, K.; White, K.W.; Pals, J.L. Continuity and Change in the Life Story: A Longitudinal Study of Autobiographical Memories in Emerging Adulthood. *J. Personal.* **2006**, *74*, 1371–1400. [CrossRef]
37. Schechter, M.; Herbstman, B.; Ronningstam, E.; Goldblatt, M.J. Emerging Adults, Identity Development, and Suicidality: Implications for Psychoanalytic Psychotherapy. *Psychoanal. Study Child.* **2018**, *71*, 20–39. [CrossRef]
38. Pasupathi, M.; Weeks, T.L. Integrating self and experience in narrative as a route to adolescent identity construction. *New Dir. Child. Adolesc. Dev.* **2011**, *2011*, 31–43. [CrossRef] [PubMed]
39. Pasupathi, M.; Hoyt, T. The development of narrative identity in late adolescence and emergent adulthood: The continued importance of listeners. *Dev. Psychol.* **2009**, *45*, 558–574. [CrossRef] [PubMed]
40. McLean, K.C.; Mansfield, C.D. The co-construction of adolescent narrative identity: Narrative processing as a function of adolescent age, gender, and maternal scaffolding. *Dev. Psychol.* **2012**, *48*, 436–447. [CrossRef]
41. Salvatore, G.; Dimaggio, G.; Semerari, A. A model of narrative development: Implications for understanding psychopathology and guiding therapy. *Psychol. Psychother. Theory Res. Pract.* **2004**, *77*, 231–254. [CrossRef] [PubMed]
42. Fonagy, P.; Steele, M.; Steele, H.; Moran, G.S.; Higgitt, A.C. The capacity for understanding mental states: The reflective self in parent and child and its significance for security of attachment. *Infant Ment. Health J.* **1991**, *12*, 201–218. [CrossRef]
43. Fonagy, P.; Target, M. Attachment and reflective function: Their role in self-organization. *Dev. Psychopathol.* **1997**, *9*, 679–700. [CrossRef] [PubMed]
44. Fonagy, P.; Target, M.; Gergely, G.; Allen, J.G.; Bateman, A.W. The Developmental Roots of Borderline Personality Disorder in Early Attachment Relationships: A Theory and Some Evidence. *Psychoanal. Inq.* **2003**, *23*, 412–459. [CrossRef]
45. Bowlby, J. *Attachment and Loss: Attachment*; Basic Books: New York, NY, USA, 1969; Volume I.
46. Stern, D.N.; Sander, L.W.; Nahum, J.P.; Harrison, A.M.; Lyons-Ruth, K.; Morgan, A.C.; Bruschweiler-Stern, N.; Tronick, E.Z. Non-interpretive mechanisms in psychoanalytic therapy. The "something more" than interpretation. The Process of Change Study Group. *Int. J. Psychoanal.* **1998**, *79*, 903–921.
47. Lyons-Ruth, K. The two-person unconscious: Intersubjective dialogue, enactive relational representation, and the emergence of new forms of relational organization. *Psychoanal. Inq.* **1999**, *19*, 576–617. [CrossRef]

48. Lyons-Ruth, K. The Interface Between Attachment and Intersubjectivity: Perspective from the Longitudinal Study of Disorganized Attachment. *Psychoanal. Inq.* **2007**, *26*, 595–616. [CrossRef]
49. Swann, W.B.; Read, S.J. Acquiring self-knowledge: The search for feedback that fits. *J. Personal. Soc. Psychol.* **1981**, *41*, 1119–1128. [CrossRef]
50. Swann, W.B. Identity negotiation: Where two roads meet. *J. Personal. Soc. Psychol.* **1987**, *53*, 1038–1051. [CrossRef]
51. Swann, W.B.; Bosson, J.K. Self and identity. In *Handbook of Social Psychology*; Fiske, S.T., Gilbert, D.T., Lindzey, G., Jongsma, A.E., Eds.; Wiley: Hoboken, NJ, USA, 2010; pp. 589–628. ISBN 978-0-470-13747-5.
52. Wachtel, P.L. Knowing oneself from the inside out, knowing oneself from the outside in: The "inner" and "outer" worlds and their link through action. *Psychoanal. Psychol.* **2009**, *26*, 158–170. [CrossRef]
53. Buie, D.H. Core Issues in the Treatment of Personality-Disordered Patients. *J. Am. Psychoanal. Assoc.* **2013**, *61*, 10–23. [CrossRef] [PubMed]
54. Loewald, H.W. On the therapeutic action of psycho-analysis. *Int. J. Psychoanal.* **1960**, *41*, 16–33. [PubMed]
55. Schechter, M.; Goldblatt, M. Psychodynamic therapy and the therapeutic alliance: Validation, empathy, and genuine relatedness. In *Building a Therapeutic Alliance with the Suicidal Patient*; Michel, K., Jobes, D.A., Eds.; American Psychological Association: Washington, DC, USA, 2011; pp. 93–107. ISBN 978-1-4338-0907-1.
56. Schechter, M.; Goldblatt, M.; Maltsberger, J.T. The Therapeutic Alliance and Suicide: When Words Are Not Enough: The Therapeutic Alliance and Suicide. *Br. J. Psychother.* **2013**, *29*, 315–328. [CrossRef]
57. Safran, J.D.; Crocker, P.; McMain, S.; Murray, P. Therapeutic alliance rupture as a therapy event for empirical investigation. *Psychother. Theory Res. Pract. Train.* **1990**, *27*, 154–165. [CrossRef]
58. Safran, J.D.; Muran, J.C. The resolution of ruptures in the therapeutic alliance. *J. Consult. Clin. Psychol.* **1996**, *64*, 447–458. [CrossRef]
59. Safran, J.D.; Muran, J.C.; Samstag, L.W.; Stevens, C. Repairing alliance ruptures. *Psychother. Theory Res. Pract. Train.* **2001**, *38*, 406–412. [CrossRef]
60. Kris, A.O. Helping Patients by Analyzing Self-Criticism. *J. Am. Psychoanal. Assoc.* **1990**, *38*, 605–636. [CrossRef] [PubMed]
61. Yeomans, F.E.; Clarkin, J.F.; Kernberg, O.F. *A Primer on Transference-Focused Psychotherapy for the Borderline Patient*; J. Aronson: Northvale, NJ, USA, 2002; ISBN 978-0-7657-0355-2.
62. Bateman, A.; Fonagy, P. Mentalization based treatment for borderline personality disorder. *World Psychiatry* **2010**, *9*, 11–15. [CrossRef] [PubMed]
63. Hoffman, I.Z. Dialectical thinking and therapeutic action in the psychoanalytic process. *Psychoanal. Q.* **1994**, *63*, 187–218. [CrossRef] [PubMed]
64. Goldblatt, M.J. Hostility and Suicide: The experience of aggression from within and without. In *Relating to Self-Harm and Suicide*; Briggs, S., Lemma, A., Crouch, W., Eds.; Routledge: New York, NY, USA, 2008.
65. Maltsberger, J.T.; Buie, D.H. Countertransference hate in the treatment of suicidal patients. *Arch. Gen. Psychiatry* **1974**, *30*, 625–633. [CrossRef] [PubMed]

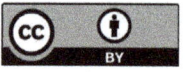

© 2019 by the authors. Licensee MDPI, Basel, Switzerland. This article is an open access article distributed under the terms and conditions of the Creative Commons Attribution (CC BY) license (http://creativecommons.org/licenses/by/4.0/).

MDPI
St. Alban-Anlage 66
4052 Basel
Switzerland
Tel. +41 61 683 77 34
Fax +41 61 302 89 18
www.mdpi.com

Medicina Editorial Office
E-mail: medicina@mdpi.com
www.mdpi.com/journal/medicina

www.ingramcontent.com/pod-product-compliance
Lightning Source LLC
LaVergne TN
LVHW070610100526
838202LV00012B/611